Reclaim Your Life After Trauma

The Power of Goal Setting

Stephanie M. Hutchins, PhD

Copyright © 2022 by Stephanie M. Hutchins

All rights reserved.

No part of this book may be reproduced, distributed, or transmitted in any form or by any means, including photocopying, recording, or other electronic or mechanical methods, without the prior written permission of the publisher, except in the case of brief quotations embodied in reviews and certain other non-commercial uses permitted by copyright law.

Dedication

To those that feel, or have felt,
that they are trapped in an inescapable cage.

Always remember that your needs matter and it's okay to make your needs a priority, even when the world tells you otherwise.
Warmest regards,
Stephanie Hutchins ♡

April 26, 2023

serotinouslife.com

Table of Contents

Introduction: Enough is Enough 7
Chapter 1: How Trauma Can Affect Your Goals 17
    You Must Want to Change 32
Chapter 2: Let's Get Specific 44
    It's All About Balance 48
    Outcome Specification 57
    What is Your Why? 65
    Digging Down Deep 68
Chapter 3: What Will People Think? 73
    Avoid the Soul-Suckers 80
    It's Time to Get Angry 87
    Be Careful of Your Ego 91
Chapter 4: Destructive Habits and Limiting Beliefs 96
    The Power of Reframing 110
    Be Kind to Yourself 125
Chapter 5: Taking Action 127
    Getting Started 130
    Building Momentum 141
    Looming Deadlines 146
    Routines and Accountability 150
Chapter 6: Continuous Improvement 158
    Tame Your Inner Critic 167
    Fill Your Mind With Positivity 180
Chapter 7: Ask for Help 189
Conclusion: Enjoy the Journey 201
Acknowledgments 206
End Notes 208

Introduction

Enough is Enough

It's around 10:00 pm on May 27, 2009, and I'm staring at myself naked in front of my full-length mirror. My long, curly brown hair is wild and frizzy from the hours I've spent obsessively trimming out its split ends. I can see the red marks on my arms and legs from picking at the bumps and other imperfections on my skin. I stare at the red stretch marks sprawled across my stomach after gaining 50 pounds during the past year. I lifted my arm and smelled the stench coming from my pits. How long has it been since I last showered? How long has it been since I've left the house? Let's see... Mom was here on Saturday, and today is—what day is it actually?

I stepped away from the mirror to find my phone; it was on the nightstand next to my bed. I sat down on the bed and soon realized I hadn't showered or left the house for four days! No wonder I look and smell so terrible. I lay back in my bed reflecting on the conversation with my mother four days earlier. We were sitting on the couch in my living room when she gave me an ultimatum. "Either you get help, or I won't keep supporting you financially," she said. Mom had had enough of watching me self-destruct. She told me to set up an appointment with a therapist that my sister, Christina, found. She also told me to put my house up for sale, which I've only owned for a little over a year.

I sigh as I think about my house. I'm so lonely here. Everywhere I look, I think about the plans that Stan and I had for this house. We were going to make it our home, but now, that could never be possible. I thought about what it felt like to feel his cold body when I found him dead on the floor of his home a week and a half before I closed on this house. My mind drifted to all the strange men I had recently had in my bed, trying to replicate what I had lost after Stan died. Then I thought, "Maybe tonight should be the night that I kill myself?"

My cat, Molly, jumped up on the bed. How interesting that she would come onto the bed at this very moment. I can't count the number of times I had decided not to kill myself because I was worried that she and my other cat, Sophie, would go hungry and eat me. I drifted off to sleep.

I woke up the next morning, fed the cats, and decided to shower. I stood there in the shower for a long time, letting the warm water run over me, cleansing the filth from my body. As the water ran down my body, I envisioned it washing my pain away. When I got out of the shower, I stared at my face in the bathroom mirror and said, "Enough is enough, Stephanie. Mom is right. This has to stop!" I got dressed and grabbed the piece of paper Mom had left on the dining room table with the therapist's contact information. As I looked at the paper, I remembered the first therapist I saw about a year and a half before. It was a total disaster.

I decided to talk to the therapist right when I started my PhD program in January 2008. Having never talked about the traumas of my past with anyone, I found it devastating to start opening the floodgates from my past. Just a few days after I started to speak about my traumas out loud, Stan's mom found out that she had terminal cancer. She died two weeks later with Stan and me by her side. Two weeks after that, I found Stan dead. A week and a half later, I closed on the house Stan and I were supposed to move into together on the same day that I finished the first semester of my PhD program.

My life was spiraling out of control. I could barely cope. That was when my therapist gave me a book on using God to heal. I was stunned when she gave me the book. I wanted to say to her, "You mean the same God that allowed me to get violated over and over by different men?" But I didn't. I just took the book home and stared at it for a while. I eventually picked it up and flipped through the pages, but I couldn't bring myself to read it. At our next session, she asked if I liked the book, but I told her I didn't read it. I explained that although I do feel there is a higher power in the universe (a God) I have never understood how he let so many bad things happen to me. My therapist still didn't know about all my traumas. No one did.

She said, "Stephanie, unless you can learn to accept God into your life, you'll *never* heal from your traumas." I shut down after that. I don't remember anything from the appointment after that. After I left that day, I never went back.

I looked back at the piece of paper with the therapist's contact information and thought, "What if this therapist feels the same way? What then?" Then I thought about my mom's ultimatum, the collection calls, and unpaid tax bills on my kitchen table. I reminded myself, "Enough is enough, Stephanie." I made the call and set up my first appointment with my new therapist. It turned out to be one of the best calls I've ever made. My new therapist, Patricia, ended up being amazing, and I'm grateful to this day that our paths crossed.

My mom was thrilled when I called to tell her that I had made an appointment to see the therapist, but I told her I wasn't quite ready to let go of the house. Even though it was making me miserable, I felt like I would be walking away from Stan if I walked away from the house. Since I couldn't work consistently for months because of my deep depression, I told her that I was going to look for a job instead so I could pay my bills and manage the house. I ended up putting the house up for sale six months later.

Between the time of making an appointment with a therapist and putting the house up for sale, I had started teaching as an adjunct instructor at a small college. I had previous experience with delivering trainings, and as a substitute teacher in primary and secondary education classrooms, but I had never taught at the college level before. I took a semester off from my PhD program after Stan died, and I continued after that. Focusing was a big challenge for me at that time, but I was lucky my classes were online; I could do the work on the days that my sadness gave me a little reprieve. I'm so grateful that I continued with my doctoral program because that was when I met a doctoral advisor who encouraged me to teach. Teaching turned out to be a blessing during a very dark period in my life. I was still struggling with depression and suicidal thoughts, but teaching gave meaning and purpose to my life. People were impressed by me being a college instructor at only 27. They were even more impressed when I told them that I was teaching anatomy and physiology. This filled me with pride and caused my ego to inflate enough to become a life raft, so I couldn't sink down deep into the well of despair I had wallowed in for over a year.

As I grew stronger, I realized that I couldn't heal in that house, which was why I eventually decided to put it up for sale. It took me seven months to sell the house, much longer than I had hoped for. However, getting out of that house was one of the best things I could have done for myself. I made enough on the sale of the house to clear the unpaid taxes and repay my mom all the loans I took from her while at the house. I worked with my credit card companies and a debt consolidation company and paid off all the debt I had acquired while at the house. Now my life is barely recognizable. I have a great career, I'm financially secure, I have a home I love, I travel the world, and I have many loving relationships.

What will it take for you to say that you've had enough? Enough of allowing past hurts to sabotage your future success. Enough of hurting yourself because of the shame and sadness you got from your trauma. Enough of living a meaningless existence.

Sometimes it takes a push from a loved one to realize how far you've fallen, but what if that push never comes? What can you do to push yourself into change? Do you have to wait until you hit rock bottom, or can you find a way to use hope for a better future to pull you forward?

Dr. Peter Levine, founder of Somatic Experiencing said, "Trauma is about not being able to imagine a future different than the past."[1] This book will help you envision a future that's different from your past, and will provide you with tools for moving forward. That's why goal setting is the foundation of this book. Goal setting allows you to imagine a life that's different from what you're currently experiencing.

As you move through the exercises in the coming pages, I want to caution you to not focus on getting back the life you had before your trauma. This is where many people get stuck. They only focus on getting back what they've lost. When you only focus on what you've lost, it keeps you focusing on how you've been a victim, and perpetuates the idea in your mind that you'll forever be broken, and you'll never be able to move past your traumatic experiences.

After trauma, people often identify themselves by their trauma—by what they once were, or what they've lost. The coming chapters will encourage you to stop holding tight to your past so you can begin moving forward toward a future of your design.

I called my first book and my keystone coaching program *Transformation After Trauma* because that's what's possible after experiencing trauma—a *transformation*. I never want to go back to any portion of my life prior to any of my traumas, because every single aspect of my life (health, relationships, career, finances, etc.) is so much better than ever before. I realized that if I can never go back to the person I was before my trauma, then why not envision an even better version of myself moving forward?

Listening to personal and professional development audio daily changed everything for me because it interrupted negative ruminations. It also allowed me to envision a life that I hadn't previously considered before. I started to listen to stories from people who've experienced tremendous hardship and are now doing amazing things with their lives. I realized that if they could thrive after the adversity they faced, then I can too.

From my years of teaching about the human body, I know that there are minimal differences from one person to another. I know that all the people I look up to aren't special or perfect. They're just people. Again, if they can do it, so can I. That's why throughout this book I'll continue to bring up the idea of filling your mind with positive thoughts and new ways of thinking so you can break the negative thought patterns that have kept you stuck.

This book is for those individuals that are tired of the rut they're in. They're so fed up that they want to change. They can't handle one more day of the same old story they've been cycling through day in and day out.

Change requires work, and it requires giving up old ways of thinking and behaving. This is why change is difficult. Many people prefer the devil they know to the devil they don't. Although they may be frustrated with certain aspects of their lives, they still find comfort in their present routines and habits. They're uncertain of what the change will bring and the discomforts they may have to endure. So, unless they're completely fed up with their current circumstances, they aren't likely to give up the little comfort they have for the discomfort of an unknown future.

Before you can move through this book, you must know what you're hoping to get out of it. Why do you want to make a change in your life? How would your life improve if you made this change? What would your life be like if you never made a change and lived out your last days the same as you are today?

One statement I heard in the audiobook, *Success and Something Greater: Your Magic Key*, that really resonated with me was, "When you have a great pain in your life, you need a greater purpose."[2] And that's what I did. I focused on goals that were bigger than my pain. Doing this prevented me from just wallowing in my pain. It provided me with a different point of focus, one that gave meaning and purpose to my life.

Goals are important because they allow you a new way to define yourself. Instead of defining yourself by your past, your trauma, and what you did to survive in the aftermath, you can define yourself by the person you're becoming. It's why I don't like calling myself a survivor because that means I'm still defining myself by my trauma. I realize that many people find the word "survivor" empowering, and I don't want to take that sense of empowerment away from anyone. However, the word doesn't trigger a sense of empowerment in me.

People often ask me, "If you don't want to be called a survivor, what do you want to be called?" I always say, "How about an author, professor, coach, or mountaineer?" Those words fill me with pride. Why do I have to be defined by something that someone else did to me? Why do I have to be defined by something that was out of my control? I prefer to be defined by what I have within my control. I prefer to be defined by what I am now and what I am becoming.

I've always pursued my goals so feverishly after my traumas because they allowed me to define myself in new terms. Instead of being a sexual assault survivor, bulimic, and a slut, I could be a college professor, mountaineer, life coach, and author. These new terms were so much more empowering. They gave me hope that I wouldn't always be saddled by my trauma and the shame over what I did to survive in the aftermath.

Chasing a future that I designed rather than aligning with traumas that were largely out of my control has been game-changing for me. I learned that I could reinvent myself, and I've done it over and over again. When I decided that one path wasn't right for me, I charted a new path. Yes, shifting was hard, it made me doubt myself, but every shift required a new version of me. A change. A transformation. I blossomed with every pivot.

It is possible to flourish after trauma. My coaching practice, Serotinous Life, is named after serotinous cones, which only release their seeds when exposed to extreme conditions, like fire. The same applies to us; some of our greatest growth emerges from our greatest struggles. That was the primary message in my first book, *Transformation After Trauma: Embracing Post-Traumatic Growth.*

I'm a life coach. Life coaching is about helping clients to bridge the gap between where they are and where they want to be. This requires having a goal and creating a plan of action to attain that goal. This is where a journal comes in handy. It allows you to commit to your goals, and to yourself, on paper. It allows you to track your progress and evaluate areas where you may be getting stuck. If you don't already have a journal, I encourage you to get one to use as you move through this book.

Sprinkled throughout this book will be calls-to-action for you to immediately begin applying what you're learning to your life. Let's begin with your first exercise.

Activity

Get out your journal and write down the areas of your life where you've said, "Enough is enough!" What self-destructive patterns are you sick and tired of repeating? What made you pick up this book?

Trauma signifies our loss of control. The purpose of this book is to arm you with the tools to start taking your control back so you can realize that you're not shackled by your trauma and an unchangeable past. The work I'm asking you to do in this book might not always be easy, but it is important. This is your opportunity to take your power back. This book will show you how to put the reins of your life back into *your* hands. Let's begin!

Chapter 1
How Trauma Can Affect Your Goals

When I graduated high school in 2000, I was convinced I was going to be a chiropractor, and no one could persuade me otherwise. I started a bachelor's degree program in pre-chiropractic studies. In January 2002, I participated in an internship with a chiropractor who told me that I didn't need to finish my bachelors to go to chiropractic college. I could finish my prerequisite courses and directly enter the Doctor of Chiropractic degree program. I was convinced this was the best path for me because I had no doubt in my mind that being a chiropractor was what I wanted for my future career.

The college I was enrolled in would not allow me to complete the remaining courses I needed at an accelerated pace. So, within just a few weeks of receiving that nugget of information at my internship, I withdrew from the college I was enrolled in, moved back home with my mom, and started taking the remaining courses I needed for entry into a Doctor of Chiropractic program at the local State colleges. In less than a year, I applied to, was accepted by, and started my doctoral studies at one of the top chiropractic colleges in the world. Some people may be surprised at how quickly I made these decisions. The thing is, I always commit myself to my goals and act on them quickly so I don't have time to talk myself out of my decisions. Once I start moving and gaining momentum, it's hard to turn back.

I was so proud of getting accepted into what most would regard as the "best" chiropractic college in the world, and without an undergraduate degree. I was so proud that I would earn my doctorate at only 23 years old. My pride pushed me through an intense transition and an even more intense program.

Even though I took 30 credits per trimester, which was a lot, I excelled in the anatomy and physiology courses that predominated the first two years of the program. I was involved in multiple clubs and different facets of campus life. That's why it came as a surprise to my family, friends, the campus community, and even myself, when I decided to withdraw from the program after completing 6 out of 10 trimesters. I'll never forget the day I ran into one of the college administrators in the parking lot shortly after I notified the school that I was withdrawing from the program. He teared up and said, "You would have been one of the greats."

I left chiropractic college for many reasons, but the main one was that I started to experience intense back pain and bilateral sciatica (pain and numbness down the back of both legs) that I had never experienced before. I was 22 years old and was in constant pain. I had trouble sitting, standing, lying down, and walking. I couldn't stay in any position for long, and I couldn't even walk for long without my pain getting worse.

Although it was odd that I had never experienced these symptoms before, I was grateful to be under treatment at one of the world's preeminent chiropractic colleges. Back pain and sciatica are some of the conditions that chiropractors often manage in patients. I was being treated by student practitioners, who were overseen by licensed doctors of chiropractic. As my symptoms got worse, the last thing I expected was for one of the doctors in the clinic to tell me I was lying about my symptoms. The words, "I'm always honest with you. I don't know why you're not honest with me, Stephanie" are forever etched in my memory. My glimmering pride in the chiropractic profession went into a quick downward spiral after that.

I went to see another doctor outside the college's clinic, where I learned that my back pain and bilateral sciatica was due to an L5-S1 disc bulge, and I was being adjusted on the wrong side of my spine by the student practitioners at the college. Learning this was when I became fully disenchanted with the profession.

It's not surprising to me that I often doubt my intuition after I've had so many people dismiss my pleas that something wasn't right. Men telling me to ignore my feelings that something wasn't right when they were touching me as a child and teenager. Doctors telling me that I wasn't experiencing the symptoms I told them I was. Family telling me to eat when I was already full so I wouldn't offend them.

Moving swiftly after I put my mind on a goal is how I combat all the voices of people telling me not to trust my instincts. That's why I didn't waste any time moving forward once I decided to withdraw from chiropractic college mid-trimester in August 2004.

Although I was convinced that I made the right decision, I was lost for a long time after I left the college. I had so much shame when I moved back to my hometown because I felt like a failure. I was in over $80,000 of student loan debt, had completed 244 college credits, and had no degree to show for it. It about broke me when I turned 23 and knew that I wouldn't reach my goal of earning my doctorate that year. It was only a small consolation when that year, I was able to earn my Bachelor of Science degree from a college that was able to apply my credits from the various institutions I attended to a bachelor's degree without me having to take additional coursework.

People often question the strong focus I place on goal setting for moving forward after trauma. But throughout my life, I've seen how having a goal to work toward propelled me forward and kept me from moving backward. That's why I felt lost when I left chiropractic college without an alternate plan in mind. I became extremely depressed and had regular suicidal thoughts.

To avoid focusing on all that I lost and all that would never be because I left chiropractic college, I started working two to three jobs at a time for 80-90 hours per week to keep busy and fill my mind with multiple distractions. I needed this because, not only was I focusing on leaving chiropractic college, but also I was remembering the reason I needed to escape my hometown with such feverish desire in the first place.

It was in and around my hometown where I was sexually violated by 8 men between the ages of 9 and 19. That doesn't count the time I was attacked from behind at knifepoint because I was able to get away from my perpetrator. It also doesn't count the multiple times that men groped me and tried to kiss me without my consent. That was why it was impossible for me to heal in my hometown.

Once again, I had to get out of that town. I knew I had to address the traumas from my past, but I couldn't bear to talk about them. I couldn't trust the clinicians in or around my hometown to keep my privacy, so I felt I needed to move away.

My sister Christina and her now husband Anthony lived in the Capital Region in New York, two hours from my hometown. I always stayed at their place to get away whenever they went out of town for the night. It felt good to be myself and get some distance from my pain. After staying there for some time, I decided to move to the capital region myself, and that's where I still live today, 15 years later.

One of the first things I did when I moved was to find a primary care doctor and get a prescription for my depression and anxiety. As expected, my new doctor encouraged me to seek therapy in addition to taking the medication. However, I told her I wasn't ready yet. I could barely cope with my current life, so how could I cope with going into the traumatic past which I had locked away in a separate compartment in the deepest recesses of my being, so I could pretend that they never happened?

It took some trial and error to find a medication that worked well for me, but over time I started to feel better. I liked my new apartment and took regular walks around the neighborhood. That apartment complex is where I met Stan. Even though my life shattered to pieces after he died, he provided me with a glimmer of hope. He also implanted the seed of belief in me that I am lovable and deserve respect and kindness.

Some people may think that I regret my decision to start a doctor of chiropractic program without finishing my bachelor's degree, or my decision to leave chiropractic college when I only had a little over a year to finish the program, but I don't regret either. Even though my life fell apart after I left chiropractic college, it all worked out for the best. Even though I was committed to the chiropractic philosophy that our body has the innate wisdom to heal itself, I had a difficult time practicing the manual adjustments. I was so afraid of hurting the person I was touching. Most people who had ever touched me had hurt me, so I wasn't sure I could touch someone without hurting them.

I withdrew from chiropractic college right before I was ready to start working in the clinic and practicing on patients. There is no doubt that I was disenchanted by the experiences I had in the clinic, but part of me wonders if I was subconsciously looking for a way to leave chiropractic college so I didn't have to touch patients.

I completed my 200-hour yoga teacher training 15 years after I left chiropractic college. Learning to assist fellow students deeper into a yoga pose brought up a lot of emotions for me, particularly from chiropractic college. I was still very uncomfortable touching people. I still didn't trust my hands and abilities.

By the time I started my yoga teacher training, I was in a much better place to go inward and start thinking about my past. I spent time reflecting on my traumas and how they still affect me today. I never thought about my traumas when I was in chiropractic college because I pretended they never happened. So, I wasn't able to put together my difficulty in doing manual adjustments with me being hurt by the hands of others. It wasn't until after I started my yoga teacher training that I began sifting through my old journals and poems to write my first book. It wasn't until I read through years of memories that I counted for the first time just how many pairs of hands had hurt me.

When I realized just how many men had hurt me and how old I was when the abuses started, it made me realize that my traumas are also why I have such difficulty being around children. I don't trust myself around them. I know I would never hurt them sexually, but I do worry about hurting them physically or emotionally. I get so anxious around them that I worry that I won't be able to control my emotions and what I would do around them if I were to get upset.

For as long as I can remember, I've said that I never wanted to have children. I was so scared of hurting them or failing them in some way. However, when I was 35, my boyfriend at the time and I tried to get pregnant. We tried for a year but it never happened. We both were tested by a fertility doctor, and the doctor couldn't find anything to explain why I wasn't getting pregnant. Given what I know about how anxiety and stress can impact our bodies, I'm certain that the sheer overwhelm I had felt at the prospect of hurting a child—my child—was too much for my body to handle.

Now that I am 39, and 40 is right around the corner, I still wonder what my life would have been like if I was able to have a child. Even though I'm scared around children, I'm actually good with them, and most children enjoy being around me. Part of me feels a pang of sadness and loss when I think that my trauma could have resulted in me missing out on the opportunity to have children. I manage to combat that emotion by thinking of ways I'll leave a legacy and give back to the world now that I won't have a child left behind after I'm gone.

I now see my books as my legacy. I see the influence I can have on my stepdaughter, my four nieces, and nephew as another way to leave my mark before it's time to exit this world. I use a similar tactic when thinking about my decision to leave chiropractic college when part of it was likely due to my past trauma. I was able to apply credits from my doctor of chiropractic program to the bachelors, masters, and doctoral degrees I ultimately did earn. I went on to teach anatomy and physiology at the college level with what I learned in chiropractic college. I was a great teacher, who impacted the lives of many students. Now I use what I know about the human body and mind to help myself and others move forward after trauma.

Although I never anticipated how my traumas would affect my choice of career and my desire to have children, I wasn't surprised by how my traumas impacted my relationship with myself and others. From years of having multiple abusers remind me that all I was good for was how my body could be used to serve them, I developed a deep sense of self-loathing. I felt I was unlovable and nothing I did was ever good enough. To combat these feelings, I became an overfunctioner. I stuffed all my pain and sadness down inside me where they couldn't be easily accessed. I hid my feelings from others. I wanted so much to please those in my life and never wanted my discomfort to become their discomfort. I became as independent as possible, so I would never be needy. This served two purposes; I didn't put undue pressure on those around me and therefore I wasn't a burden, and I didn't get too close to people or depend on anyone so I wouldn't get hurt.

I aimed to excel at everything so I could be looked at as good or significant. The men who abused me constantly reminded me how insignificant I was. They used me and discarded me as though I was disposable. My accomplishments in school and ultimately in my career became a way to get noticed. The more recognition I got for my accomplishments, the more I wanted to achieve. Unfortunately, this led to me forming a strong attachment to many things, especially titles and money. I've always felt that these things dictate who I am. So if I let them all go, who will I be? Will I like that person hiding behind the facade? I was never sure.

Although I'm better at controlling my ego today, I'm still very proud of my accomplishments. I understand that a certain level of pride is acceptable. I worked hard for what I've achieved. But I know deep down that I still attach my accomplishments and financial holdings to my self-worth. I also learned to become a great storyteller and captivate the attention of my audience. I always wanted to be the most interesting person in the room.

I don't want to condemn these coping mechanisms because they served me in many ways. Not only did they help to combat the self-loathing and lack of self-worth, but they also resulted in me achieving great success in my academic studies and career. However, they came with a cost. Today I'm a little better at my ego not getting the better of me, but that's only because I don't need it as much as I used to. I mentioned earlier in this book that my ego served as a life raft for me when I was experiencing immense pain. Now that I'm safely on land, I don't have the need to jump in that life raft as often.

Unfortunately, the effects of my trauma still linger, as they always will. In intimate relationships, I still need constant reminders that my partner loves me and that I matter to him. I'm still highly sensitive to being ignored. Watching my partner scrolling through his phone while I'm talking still triggers me; it signals that what I'm saying doesn't matter, and that I don't matter. I still get upset if my partner doesn't want to touch me because I feel like something is wrong with me, and my body is too disgusting to touch.

This feeling that my body is repulsive led me into a severe eating disorder. At its worst, I would binge and purge 8-12 times per day. Even though my bulimia is considered to be in remission because I haven't purged in years, I still eat until my stomach hurts from time-to-time. I also must be careful of how I look at my body. I was categorized as being morbidly obese in my late 20s. Now in my late 30s, I'm at a normal weight, but I still have extra skin, wrinkles, and cellulite from the extra weight I used to carry. Now whenever I start to look at myself in the mirror with disgust, I must remind myself to thank my body for all that it's done for me.

The deep-rooted feelings of unworthiness and disgust about my body led me into being extremely promiscuous. Not only that, but my trauma also attracted me to the same type of men that continued to hurt me. So, not only did I sleep with a lot of men, but I slept with a lot of men that didn't care about me and saw my body simply as a vessel for their pleasure. This is interesting considering that I slept with more men than I dare to count, all in an effort to prove that my body was okay to touch. However, I ended up choosing men that probably would have touched anybody that would have given them even a moment of pleasure.

Fortunately, the promiscuity has passed. I now have a greater love and respect for my body and I'm more comfortable in my skin. I still must be careful of not falling into old cycles with the men that I date. As I continue to heal, the men I choose become less and less like the men that hurt me so long ago.

Another area the effect of my trauma still lingers today is in my friendships. I never had really close friendships until my late 30s. Being hurt by multiple people that were supposed to love me and I was supposed to trust, made me hesitant to get too close to people. However, what's interesting is that I love talking with people. I'm curious about everyone and everything, so I'm good at making quick connections with people from all backgrounds, but my MO has been to shut the relationship down the moment they want to become true friends. I would usually do this through ignoring the person's attempts to reach out. It's funny, considering that I hate when people ignore me, yet I've chosen it as a prime way to let other people know that I don't need them.

Luckily, there have been a few special women in my life that loved me anyway and have stuck by me throughout the years even though I continuously pushed them away. In the past few years, I've made a committed effort to improve the relationships with the women in my life, both friends and family, and I must say that the results have been beyond beautiful. My life has been truly enriched by my relationships. It saddens me to think about all that I missed out on by not allowing people to get close to me for my entire life up until now, but I know that I did that to protect myself. I was in so much pain and I knew that I couldn't bear the thought of enduring more. Now that I'm stronger and have more self-care practices in place to handle difficult circumstances, I'm willing to take the chance of getting hurt in an effort to experience the beauty of deep, loving relationships.

What has been interesting to experience is how I'm almost childlike in some aspects of interacting with my friends. I haven't been through all the developmental stages of friendship until now, so I'm still learning how to navigate certain aspects of friendship. Now, my greatest fear in my friendships is being left, or them saying they don't want me in their life anymore.

I'm figuring out how to navigate sharing some of my thoughts, feelings, and criticisms with my friends without hurting them. Probably one of the best examples of this is when I was on a hike with my friend, Teri. I usually let others take the lead in hikes but I must follow close behind the person in front of me so I can hear them. The multiple ear infections I had as a child damaged my hearing. I actually qualify for hearing aids, and I realize it's vanity that's stopping me from getting the hearing aids. Until I decide to relinquish and get the hearing aids, I continue to find ways to navigate around my hearing loss.

So on hikes, I follow close behind my hiking partners so I can hear what they're saying. When my friend, Teri, started using hiking poles, I noticed that she liked to primarily use one pole and keep the other one pointed behind her. I tried my best to stay further behind her, but with my difficulty in hearing, I kept creeping closer to her. This didn't become a big deal until we began climbing uphill. At that point, I was at risk of losing an eye if I got too close.

Instead of saying anything, I just kept trying to monitor my distance from her. But the continual concern over losing an eye caused me to stop dead in my tracks and say, "Teri, I have to tell you something." She was surprised and said, "Of course, what is it?" I proceeded to tell her that I was concerned about losing an eye and asked her if she could stop holding her pole behind her. She of course had no idea she even held her pole that way and I was at risk of losing an eye. So, she asked why I didn't tell her sooner. I told her I worried about upsetting her. To her surprise and mine, I began to cry. I told her I was so worried that she wouldn't hike with me again. She was so sweet and hugged me. She reassured me that it was no big deal, and of course she will hike with me again, and to let her know whenever she holds her pole like that again.

Later in the day, I explained that I never learned how to be a friend and how to set boundaries in a friendship. I felt so silly saying these things as a 39-year-old woman. I've spent my life trying to navigate the emotions of others, trying my best to never make myself a burden, and trying to never let my needs take over theirs. Since that time, it's been easier for me to share similar types of criticisms with other friends without crying. However, I usually come to a dead stop in the same way I did with Teri on the hiking trail and prepare them for what I think will likely shatter our friendship, usually to just have them shrug it off like it was no big deal. I believe they don't really categorize what I'm saying as a criticism. They just see it as feedback and me expressing my feelings. However, what's different for me is that I consider all feedback a criticism.

I realize that much of these concerns over sharing criticisms of my friends with them are a projection of how uncomfortable I am with being criticized. I have a very difficult time with being criticized. I take every criticism as evidence of how I am no good. It's why I looked at very few student reviews during my 12 years as a college professor, and today I stop myself from looking at reviews on my first book. 95% of the reviews could be glowing, yet I'll ruminate over the one or two that are negative. I still have more work to do in this aspect of my life. I try my hardest to look at criticism with objectivity and view it as helpful feedback going forward. However, this feeling that I am no good is a core belief. This destructive belief could take years to excavate, but I continue to find ways to navigate around it so it doesn't hold me back from reaching my goals.

This feeling of not being good enough is shared by many people, even those who haven't experienced trauma. Society tells us all in a myriad of ways that we're not good enough so we'll buy what they're selling—a diet pill that will help us drop some pounds; clothes that will accentuate our features; skincare products that will revitalize our skin; scents that will allow us to attract the opposite sex; the house, car, or doodad that will make us feel that we have a higher status in society. Trauma just exacerbates what society already tells us.

Trauma can also destroy our confidence. It can cause us to doubt ourselves at every turn. Although trauma can affect our confidence, it's normal to doubt ourselves and our abilities. Even people who haven't experienced trauma doubt themselves sometimes. Doubt is a way that our brain protects us from getting hurt, but it can also prevent us from experiencing all that life has to offer. Just because trauma can make building confidence more difficult, it doesn't make it impossible.

Activity

Get out your journal and write down the ways your trauma has affected your life. This activity is not meant for you to wallow in your pain. Instead of immersing yourself in the feelings associated with your trauma and the ways that it's impacted your life, look at the aftermath as an objective observer. Try to get some distance from it.

If someone was looking at you and your life since your trauma, how would they view how the trauma has impacted you, your relationships, career, financial situation, etc.?

If you begin to feel overwhelmed at any point during this activity, sit back, take a few deep breaths, and continue. If you're still too overwhelmed to continue, you can walk away and come back to it at another time.

The purpose of this activity is not to bring you into your pain, it's to look at it as an outsider and see how your trauma has affected your decisions. This awareness is the first step in breaking patterns in the future that you no longer want to repeat.

This activity is also not about making you upset over all that you've lost and all that will no longer be because of your trauma. After you identify areas of your life where trauma has affected you, I want you to also identify something positive that came from it. We'll revisit this again in Chapter 4, but I want you to start now with thinking about what you've gained from your trauma. I know it may seem difficult, especially if your trauma led you to self-destructive habits or abusive relationships, but if you look hard enough, there is positive in every situation. By beginning to look at your painful experiences differently, you'll begin to release the hold those experiences have over you.

We'll never fully break free from our trauma. We'll always be a work in progress. But that's good! That means we'll always have opportunities for growth and change. I feel like I've lived many different lives because, over time I'm continually transforming into a different version of myself. Our opportunity for growth is directly proportional to the amount of pain we've experienced. The more pain, the more opportunity for growth.

Even though I've done an immense amount of healing, I continue expanding my ability for growth by expanding my goals. Now that my pain is diminishing, my opportunity for growth is directly proportional to the size of my goals. The bigger my goals, the greater my opportunity for continued growth.

I used goal setting to get through my pain and I continue to use goal setting to move beyond my pain. What this has given me is a way to continually transform myself. Each time I become a different version of myself, I experience life in new and more beautiful ways.

You Must Want to Change

I'm often asked in interviews what it takes to move forward after trauma. The first thing I always say is: "The person must want to change." Most people look at me with a perplexed look when I say this, as they assume that people who've been depressed, unable to work, or harming themselves in a variety of ways, must want to change. But this isn't always the case. Sometimes there is one part of the person that wants to change while another part of them is in conflict and doesn't want to change.

Some people don't want to change because they've given up hope and feel that life can never get better. And because they've given up hope, they don't even see a point in trying to change their life circumstances. Unfortunately, when a person has reached this place, they're not likely going to be receptive to new ideas that could break their destructive thought patterns. These individuals are unlikely to read this book or others like it. If they do, they'll continually look at it with a critical lens, finding fault throughout the pages, and identify all the ways in which the content doesn't apply to them.

For these people, there's usually nothing anyone can do to talk them out of it. It's sad, disappointing, and you want to take them and shake them and say, "Change is possible!" This effort will, unfortunately, be wasted if they're not ready to receive that information. I understand this place of complete darkness, devoid of all hope. I fell into a deep depression in my mid-20s. I contemplated suicide on an almost daily basis because I just never thought life could get any better. I understand that people can get to that point, and it's not always possible for someone else to help them reach that place where they want to turn things around.

You can't force somebody to change. That's why it often takes people who get into this mindset to reach rock bottom—a place of extreme pain and misery—before they'll make the decision to change. When my mom gave me the ultimatum that I get help or she'll stop supporting me financially, I was already at rock bottom. I knew if I continued on the path I was on, I would die.

If you have a loved one in that place where they've lost all hope, I understand how difficult this must be for you. Please know that I'm not saying you should give up on them. It was through the love of my mother, her belief that I could change, and watching for glimmers of hope in me, that she was able to help me turn the corner. When later discussing with my mother, her decision to set a firm boundary with me and tell me she wasn't going to continue to support me financially, she of course expressed how difficult the decision was for her. However, she felt that there was a part of me that was ready to change. She also knew that previous attempts to help were not making any difference, and she was concerned that they might have been making things worse. It turned out that the best thing she could have done to help was to stop helping me.

If you're ever in a similar situation as my mother was with me, please don't give up on your loved one. Know that it's going to be difficult for them to turn that corner. Sometimes it may take finding hope. That hope may come from spiritual or religious experiences. That hope may come from reading or listening to a story that's similar to theirs. Sometimes it may be hitting rock bottom, or it may be a combination of hitting rock bottom and experiencing a glimmer of hope.

It'll be devastating to watch your loved one go down a path of self-destruction that could lead to their death. You'll feel helpless, and at times you may feel as hopeless as your loved one. You must do things to protect yourself during this painful time. You can use a variety of tools to take care of yourself—spiritual or religious practices, connections with family and friends, talking to a counselor or participating in group counseling sessions with people in similar circumstances, getting regular sleep and exercise, and eating a healthy diet.

If you've experienced extreme heartache in life and are taking the time and energy to read this book and do the activities, and you find yourself connecting with these words, then there is a part of you that is ready to change and has hope that change is possible.

But if there's a part of you that continually thinks that what you're reading isn't possible, then there's a part of you that doesn't want to change and feels that change isn't possible. The following paragraphs and activities will help you evaluate the part of you that doesn't want to change.

It's often difficult for people to understand that every behavior or habit they have exists because it's served them in some way. It's hard to give something up if it serves us, even if it does create challenges for us. Now what I'm going to write next might be hard to read, but it's important to think about. Please remember what I've shared about my trauma. I understand how difficult it can be to not only experience the trauma but to learn to accept and forgive the person you become after your trauma. Please know that I mean absolutely no harm in anything I write. So please sit back and take a deep breath before I share the next activity with you.

Part of the work you'll be doing in the next activity is answering the question: "What are you gaining by holding onto your trauma?" In other words, "What are you gaining by remaining a victim?" Now, I know you might want to get angry at me for even suggesting such a thing, but please hear me out. If you previously felt starved for attention and after your trauma you received more sympathy and attention than you ever have before, you're going to be less likely to give up being a victim. At least, right now. Please know there's no shame in that. You don't need to feel ashamed by wanting attention. Feeling significant is a basic human need, and sometimes our traumas allow us to appear more significant to those that previously ignored us. Even if you think you might be struggling with this, keep moving through this book. You can't change something unless you're first aware of it.

Let me reiterate, there's absolutely nothing to be ashamed of if you discover that you've been gaining some benefits by remaining a victim after your trauma. Many of us who've experienced trauma have a lifetime of hurts that occurred before the trauma and likely occurred afterward as well. For some of us, the most attention we received in our whole lives was after being traumatized and others knowing about it. So, if you've always struggled with feeling insignificant and unimportant, it's not surprising you're going to hold on to the one thing that has gotten you the attention you've always craved.

Again, feeling significant is a basic human need and it's very normal. However, it's important to become aware of the benefit you may still be gaining by not moving past your trauma. You must know that you're in complete control of your life's journey, even after your trauma. Regardless, if there's one part of you that wants to move past your trauma, and another part that doesn't, you'll likely keep getting tripped up in the process. That's why it's important to acknowledge the part of you that's in conflict with your desire to heal, and move past some of the worst experiences of your life.

In the next activity, you'll have the opportunity to evaluate any benefit you may have gained after your trauma, and why you haven't let your trauma go up to this point. I recognize that this will be a challenging exercise. So, you can step away and pick it back up when you're ready. I know it could be very scary to write that you appreciated and enjoyed the attention and recognition that you received after your trauma. I can't remind you enough that this isn't about shaming yourself or developing an even deeper sense of self-hatred for yourself. You can't change something unless you're first aware of it. This is about bringing that part of you to the forefront that's trying to fill that empty void inside of you where that feeling of insignificance lies.

Some of us are in relationships where we're not appreciated. Why do we get upset when our significant other doesn't say thank you or recognize the work we do? Because we want to feel significant. Why is it hard when our children leave home and don't need us anymore? It's because we used to be significant and now we're not anymore. Why is it hard for us at our jobs to not be appreciated and recognized for the good work we do?

We want to feel significant because it's a basic human need. When we've been deprived of that feeling of significance in all the different aspects of our life, and then all of a sudden we're showered with recognition, significance, and sympathy after our traumatic event, an empty void is being filled inside of us. It's no wonder that part of us wants to hold onto it and not let go.

Now take a deep breath and let's move onto the next activity. It's time to acknowledge the part of you that doesn't want to let go of being a victim. As I previously said, there's nothing to be ashamed of if there is a part of you that wants to hold onto the hurt and pain that your trauma has caused you. It's about taking your power back. Once you see that there's part of you that could be sabotaging your efforts to move past your trauma, you can begin to change it. You can't change something if you're not aware that you're doing it or that it's a problem. Awareness is the key to making any change!

Tony Robbins identifies six basic human needs; certainty, uncertainty/variety, significance, connection/love, growth, and contribution.[3] I've found that most people hold onto their trauma because it gives them a feeling of significance. I've based much of this section on the assumption that your trauma also provides *you* with the feeling of significance. However, if you feel that this isn't true and that another basic human need is being met, please address that instead in the coming questions.

Here we go. This might be hard, but it's okay. You'll get through it. If at any point this becomes difficult, sit back, take a few deep breaths, walk away if you need to, and then come back to it.

Activity

Get out your journal and write down what you're gaining by holding onto your trauma. What empty space in your life is it filling? Then write about what caused this empty space to develop.

After you're done writing, acknowledge this part of you that wants to hold onto the trauma and any benefits being a victim has provided you. Can you feel where the emptiness is inside your body? Is it in your mind? Is it in your heart? Is it in your belly? Sit back, close your eyes, and really sense what part of your body feels a sense of emptiness. Place your hands on that area and while keeping your eyes closed, thank that part of you for trying to protect you and make you whole. It's important to understand that your mind and body are trying to hold onto this negativity for a reason. So, thank this part of you for its work in trying to help you, and tell it that you're ready to let go of this pain so you can replace it with something even better.

You can't just remove one way of thinking without replacing it with another. You can't change a bad habit without replacing it with a better one. So that means if significance is something you're gaining from your trauma, you may not be ready to let go of the trauma until you have something else to obtain that feeling of significance from. That's why the next activity will ask you to brainstorm ideas for how you can fill the void you just identified so that your trauma doesn't have to live there any longer.

In preparation for the next activity, ask yourself: "If I don't feel significant and my trauma gives me that sense of significance by people paying attention to me, what can I replace that with?" In what other ways can you gain recognition and the feeling of significance so that your body and mind won't keep holding onto the trauma to fill that gap? Can you volunteer? If so, what types of organizations would give you the greatest sense of purpose? Can you take on a new project at work where your skills will really shine? Are you creative? Do you like to paint, draw, write, play music, or sing? If so, can you work on your art and sell it, or start posting it on social media to have people commend you for your talent? Are you athletic? If so, can you start engaging in different competitions like 5K's, triathlons, or a different type of competition to get recognized for your talent?

Social media has its issues, but one thing it's great at is providing people with a feeling of significance. When we get likes and comments, we feel significant. So if you get recognized for something at work, you completed a creative project, or competed in an athletic competition, you could tell your social media followers about it. However, you must know that you don't need others to validate yourself and your work. Just the mere practice of engaging in something that makes you feel good and fills you with personal pride, is enough. The external validation helps some people make their internal beliefs a little stronger if confidence is lacking initially. Over time, you'll begin to build enough belief and confidence in yourself that your need for external validation will minimize over time and you'll be able to get that feeling of significance simply by you knowing that you did a good job. However, it can take time to get there.

If you've been oppressed by others during a significant portion of your life, it might be challenging for you to start coming up with ways you can feel significant because you might not feel good at anything. Please don't worry, start small. This is where the important work of building up your confidence will come in. Later in this book, I'll provide you with ideas of how to start building up your belief in yourself and what you're good at. My hope is that one step at a time you'll realize your strength, inner beauty, and talents. I don't believe that any of us entered this world empty without gifts or talents, it just takes time to study *you* to get a better understanding and appreciation of what you have to offer.

Once you're able to gain significance in another aspect of your life, it's going to be easier to let go of your trauma. Don't get discouraged if this process takes a while, especially if a lack of confidence is an issue. I promise you, just the mere fact that you're now aware that part of you wants to hold onto your trauma will be life changing. It'll allow you to start interrupting that cycle of looping back into the past and tapping into your trauma to fill a void inside of you. You'll be able to look at that part of yourself, acknowledge the work it's trying to do to fill a void, and kindly tell that part of you, "Thank you, but I don't need you anymore."

I know it might seem a little silly to talk to yourself, but it's actually very important. We have so much internal chatter going on inside our minds constantly that we need to learn to tell our minds to, "Quiet down." If you haven't already, I encourage you to read my book, *Transformation After Trauma: Embracing Post-Traumatic Growth*, which is filled with a variety of self-care tools. Self-care practices like meditation are helpful in learning ways to move past self-defeating internal chatter.

Even if you don't believe that holding onto your trauma is filling the need of significance, significance is still a basic human need. So, still work on ways that you can begin to expand on your feeling of significance. It'll help to build your confidence and belief in yourself and your abilities. This will help you achieve other goals in your life and propel you further from your trauma.

If you're having a difficult time with this, start by making a list of times when you've been commended or congratulated by anyone before. Dig deep into your past if you need to. Maybe it was a family member, a friend, a colleague, a boss, or a teacher. Did they recognize you for your kindness, how well you did on an exam, how great of a job you did on a work project, or how much they appreciated you listening when they were upset? It doesn't matter what they acknowledged you for, just write it down. A trend might begin to appear. You might start to notice that different people have acknowledged your talents or strengths in the same area. This might start to create ideas in your mind about what you can start pursuing that will give you the recognition or feeling of significance that you're looking for.

If you're still having difficulty finding examples, then start being mindful each day from here on out about when somebody recognizes you for anything good about you or something you did. Keep a piece of paper and pen with you or use a note-taking app on your phone to keep a running list. Write examples down as soon as you receive a compliment. As you start writing things down, you'll likely start remembering times in your past when you've been complimented for similar things.

Activity

Get out your journal and first write down what you can do to fill the gap created by your life circumstances so your trauma doesn't need to continue to fill that void. Then, write down the actions you can start taking *today* to begin filling this gap. For example, if you decide to volunteer, you can begin with researching organizations in your area that you can serve in. If you decide to engage in an athletic competition, you can begin researching upcoming competitions in your area. If you decide to paint, start with picking up your paint brush today!

You must also be receptive to new ways of thinking. To stop recycling the same thought processes over and over, you must be ready to accept new ways of thinking so you can begin new thought processes. This is why I regularly bring up how important personal development is to me. Reading books, listening to audio through podcasts, YouTube, or audio books, and going to workshops have all been immensely helpful in changing my mindset. They input new ways of thinking into my mind when I'm ready to receive the information. Sometimes I take a break and come back to it and read or listen again and again, and each time I pursue new information and new ways of thinking, some part of me always changes. Sometimes in big ways and sometimes small, but over time, the changes add up to enormous shifts, and ultimately transformation.

Even if you're not fully there yet, I know some part of you is ready to start making a shift in your life, otherwise you wouldn't have started reading this book. So even if part of you is hesitant to fully commit yourself to change, honor the part of you that does by continuing to read on. Maybe something will cause a shift in your mindset and a bigger part of you will desire change. You have the option to continue to experience life the way you are, and you also have the option to choose to experience life in a new way.

I'm in complete agreement with the popular quote from former United States Secretary of State, Condoleezza Rice: "I firmly believe you never should spend your time being the former anything." So, I encourage you to consider how your life would change for the better if you were to leave the comfort zone of your present story. You can change your story at any moment you choose. You can change what your pain means to you. You have the choice to pivot and move in a different direction at any point you choose. My hope is that the coming chapters will inspire you to open yourself up to new ways of thinking and to try the tools provided to begin making movement toward a new life.

Chapter 2

Let's Get Specific

After falling so far after Stan died, it was hard to know where to begin when I started to pick up the pieces of my life and put them back together. It was a long, arduous process, but bit by bit, I got stronger as I aimed for one goal and then another. Some of the earliest steps were the hardest. I had fallen into such a deep hole that I wasn't showing myself any self-care or self-love because I didn't feel that I deserved it.

After I said "Enough is enough" and decided to change, some of the hardest things for me were to start brushing my teeth, bathing myself, and cleaning my home because I didn't think I was worth even basic forms of self-love. All I could focus on was how bad of a person I must be to have all these things happen to me. It was hard to show myself even the slightest form of love and compassion, so starting with cleaning myself and my home were important first steps.

I experienced so much degradation from man after man using me for what they wanted. Many told me I was nothing and made me feel undeserving of love and affection. So why would self-love be something I would default to after years of being programmed otherwise? It wouldn't be. So it took a lot of effort to begin taking care of myself again in some of the simplest ways. That means I had to do these things even though I didn't feel worthy. This is where people often get tripped up in the goal setting process. They think they must wait until they feel ready, until they have the confidence, or until they feel worthy, but that's not how it works. If you keep waiting *until*, you'll never reach your goals. You must begin working on your goals when you *don't* feel ready. Over time, you'll build momentum, confidence in yourself, and the belief that you are worthy and can achieve your goal.

Even though I didn't feel worthy at the time, I wrote down simple goals for myself each day. Literally my goals began as brushing my teeth, taking a shower, and taking out the trash. As these became habits, I no longer needed to keep writing them down. As I started to take care of myself, I started to feel better. I began writing down bigger goals, like getting a job because I hadn't been able to work regularly because of my depression. Each step made it progressively easier to do the next.

Another way that people get tripped up in the goal setting process is setting their sights on their biggest goals right away. If your goal is really big, or it's far into the future, it can feel impossible to achieve. That's why this book will cover the importance of chunking down goals into bite-sized pieces to prevent overwhelm, and build momentum. I didn't go straight into becoming a college professor, completing my PhD, climbing mountains, and traveling around the world. I went one step at a time, and each step made it easier for me to do the next.

The next goal in line after looking for a job was to stop sleeping with so many strange men. This took some time, but I was able to stop this by keeping around a few men consistently for casual sex. I told myself that I must be good, significant, and enough if they kept coming back. Luckily, this need to have sex with a man to prove my worth has diminished.

After successfully ending the meaningless sex, I moved onto losing weight. At 5 foot 4 inches tall and 222 pounds, I was classified as morbidly obese. I had sleep apnea and high cholesterol, and I wasn't even 30 years old yet. Food is my one great love and my preferred form of self-destruction, and I wasn't ready to give it up just yet, so I turned to exercise. It was a natural choice as I've always loved to exercise, particularly outdoors. I've always loved to walk and enjoy being in nature, so I began looking for Meetup groups that would allow me the opportunity to socialize and be active at the same time.

I found a number of hiking groups to participate in. It was hard to keep up with many of the groups because I hadn't exercised consistently for years and I was carrying many pounds of excess weight. So I began to look for hikes that I could do on my own. This way, I wouldn't get nervous when I was slowing the group down. When I got nervous, I would go faster than I was capable of, tire myself out, get clumsy and trip and fall, roll my ankles, or pull muscles. I did find a hiking partner, Marv, who was able to tolerate my slow pace. We both began hiking around the same time and were both hooked once we started. For a few years, we hiked almost every weekend together. I trusted him and felt safe with him. Between the mountains Marv and I hiked together, and the ones I hiked by myself, I was hiking over 100 mountains each year for several years in a row.

The mountains were the perfect healing ground for me. In the beginning of my hiking, I wanted to give up on almost every hike, but I didn't. I kept going even though I was tired and sore. Each time I persevered toward my goal—the summit—even though I was uncomfortable, I proved to myself how strong I was. Each time I pushed through the discomfort and reached my goal, I felt a greater sense of pride in myself, and my confidence in myself began to soar.

As my body got stronger with each hike, I began to set my sights on bigger hikes and climbs around the United States and the world. I have since climbed all the 4,000 foot mountains in the Northeastern US, 39 of the 50 US State highpoints, the highest point in Central America, the highest point in Europe, and the highest point in Africa.

As Benjamin Hardy said in *Personality Isn't Permanent*, "In order to become a new person, you must have a new goal—a purpose worth pursuing."[4] It's so easy to keep cycling through the past after trauma. But setting goals and creating a plan to move toward those goals helps you create a way out which means there's hope. Goal setting was hands down *the most* important part of my healing journey, and I believe it'll also be the most important part of *your* healing journey.

Setting goals gives you hope that your future reality can be better than your past or present reality. As Les Brown said, "If you don't know what your goal is right now, don't worry, just make something up and write that down. You gotta have something you're aiming at. People aiming at nothing in life end up hitting nothing dead on the head."[5] As you start experiencing initial wins, it'll help build confidence in yourself to achieve even bigger goals and encourage you to keep exploring what's possible.

This is where you begin taking a hold of the reins of your life and start determining the direction that you want your life to go. In the coming activities, you'll have the opportunity to examine where you are now in your life in relation to where you want to be. This is not about being hard on yourself for not being farther along, or to get caught up in how hard it'll be to reach the kind of life you desire. This is the opportunity for you to start to think about what's important to you in your life. What makes you happiest? What does being happy even look like to you?

Trauma can be so devastating because of the loss of control we had over our circumstances at the time. After traumatic experiences, it becomes easy to think that if we didn't have control then, that we don't really have control over anything in our lives. However, this is where you have the opportunity to start challenging that belief.

Use the work you'll be doing in this book to start pushing those limitations you believe you have, and start dreaming. Yes, this world can be a dark, scary place at times, but it can also be vibrant and beautiful. This is your opportunity to see that your trauma is over, and you can start crafting your plan for moving past it.

It's All About Balance

Trauma overwhelms one's ability to cope. Throughout the activities in this book, I won't ask you to dig deep into your trauma, but I'll ask you to evaluate how it's living in your life right now, even though it might be over. I want you to become aware of how your trauma is living in your body and mind, and how it's playing out in your day-to-day life.

The after-effects of trauma are so much more than what happened during the actual event. The way it plays out in our minds and bodies long after it occurred is what really wreaks havoc in our lives. We can't change anything until we understand this fact. We may understand on a very superficial level that we need to heal but we may not understand how much it's invading every aspect of our life, like our relationships, work, and finances. And that's why in the next activity, you'll evaluate every aspect of your life. Through this activity and coming activities, I'm hopeful that you'll begin to see how your trauma is stealing away your joy each day, even though your trauma is over. I'm also hopeful that you'll learn that you have the ability to choose to live a beautiful life even after hardship.

Every day, we have a choice to take our power back and stop handing over our happiness to others, especially people who don't want the job of controlling our happiness and aren't even a good fit for that job. Those of us who've experienced trauma are prone to experiencing the extremes of emotion. We tend to go full force or nothing at all. We might sleep all day, spend hours watching TV, exercise until we can't move, or work ourselves into the ground. It's understandable why we gravitate toward these extremes when we're in deep pain. During all of them, we can avoid facing the uncomfortable feelings that are inside of us, pushing them down further, hoping that ignoring them will make them go away.

It's important to recognize that you've gravitated toward these coping mechanisms for a reason. I've always gravitated toward work. I feel good when I get recognized for my work, but it's resulted in me working to extremes. There've also been points where I've exercised to extremes. Please don't misunderstand me, there's nothing wrong with working hard or pushing yourself physically. It only becomes a problem when it's taken to extremes. How do you know this? You'll know when you see that your wheel of life in the next activity has one or a few areas rating very high and others rating very low. Although my wheel has improved significantly over time, I still have a lot of room for improvement. This is the wheel of life I completed on October 20, 2021 when writing this book:

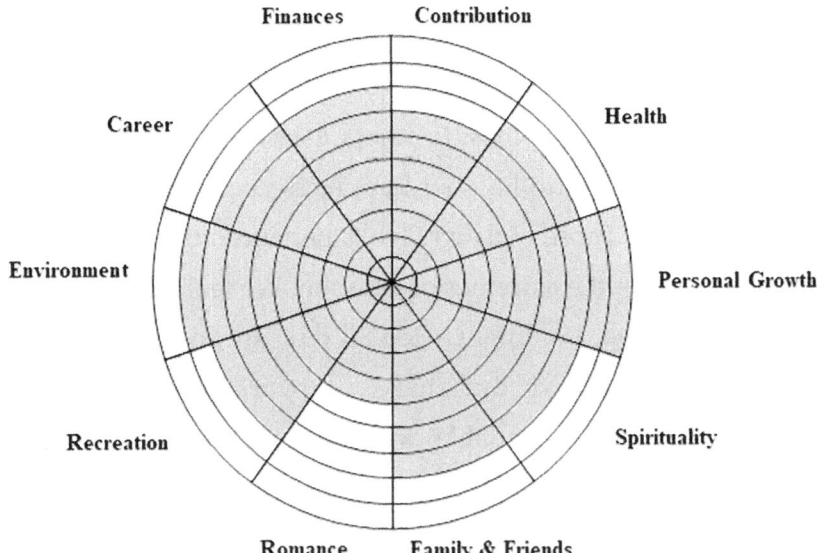

The goal of examining your wheel of life is to be able set goals that will bring all areas of your life into balance. Imagine your wheel of life as a wheel on a bicycle. If it has jagged edges, how smooth of a ride are you going to have? Not very smooth. The closer all areas of your life are to one another, the smoother your ride will be, both on the bicycle and in life. When one area of your life is low, it'll cause stress in other areas. For example, financial stress can impact your relationships and health. Relationship stressors can impact your performance at work.

From this activity, you'll be able to see the gap between where you are now and where you want to be. Bringing awareness to this gap will help keep you motivated to fill in those gaps if the process becomes challenging along the way. However, don't feel pressured to fill in a gap right away, just because you see one. For example, I currently rate my romance category as a five, and I'm single. I mark it as a five and not a zero because I'm happy being on my own, but I know that my life will be enriched by having a partner to share my life's journey with. So, I want to make progress toward finding a life partner, eventually. However, right now I have more work to do on myself before I can find a partner that I won't recycle old patterns with.

I also understand that some people don't believe that there's any such thing as a level 10 in any aspect of life, and that's okay. What you're really looking for is what areas are out of balance in your life and what you're going to do to bring those areas to the same level with others over time.

Don't overthink it. For example, for family and friends, everything might be great with everyone except one family member. Nonetheless, think of this category overall. Same applies to finances. Perhaps you're happy with what you're saving for retirement, but you still have some debts to pay off, just look at the category as a whole. Overall, how do you rate where you are now in relation to where you want to be? You'll have the opportunity to explore these areas further in coming activities.

You also don't need to find something wrong with each category. If you're completely satisfied with one area, then in the following activity, write what you're going to do to maintain that area at its current level. I marked my personal growth category as a ten, not because I have no more work to do, but because I'm so proud of how far I've come. I work on myself every day, so as long as I maintain my current personal growth habits, I'll continue to grow and change into an even better version of myself.

Furthermore, don't base your answers on anyone else changing. It can only be based on what you have control over, what you can change. If you place your happiness in someone else's hands, you might never be happy. Also, keep in mind that your wheel of life will change over time. This isn't a one and done activity. It's important to review your wheel of life every few months to see if anything has changed. Specific areas might come into balance. As you change one area of your life, other areas are bound to be affected. Your priorities might change. Maybe you previously wanted out of your relationship with your significant other, but you might find that as you work on yourself, things might naturally start to change in your relationship, and maybe you won't feel the need to leave.

Activity: Wheel of Life

It'll be easiest to complete this activity if you print out the Wheel of Life worksheet. You can access this worksheet at serotinouslife.com/worksheets. Where are you on a scale from 0 – 10 in each of these areas of your life? The middle of the circle corresponds to '0' (very dissatisfied) and the outermost ring of the circle corresponds to '10' (very satisfied). Color in each section on the chart, based on how you rate yourself in each area. You're rating yourself based on where you currently are in each area in comparison to where you really want to be. If you rate yourself a 7 in one area, you'll color in that area from 0 – 7, so you have 7 rows shaded in. Below you'll find examples of different facets of each category.

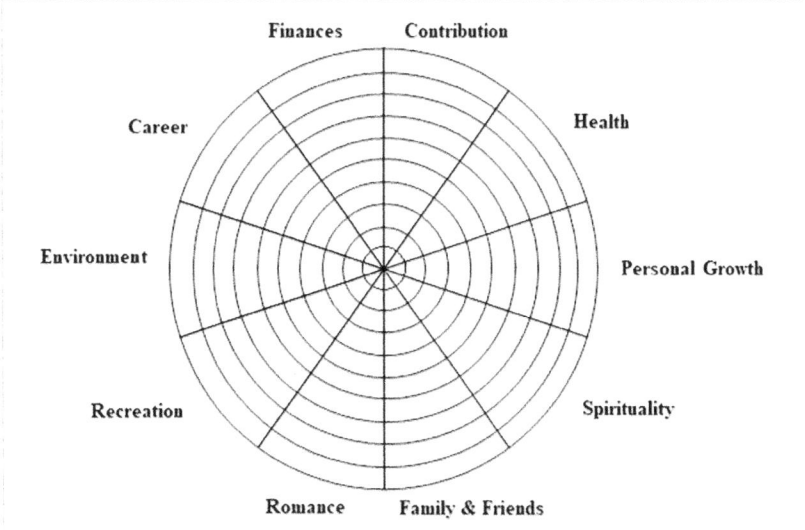

Career includes your job, business, or college studies.

Finances includes your savings, investments, retirement, and debt.

Contribution includes giving time or money to your community and causes that are important to you.

Health includes your physical body, emotional health, diet, sleep, and exercise.

Personal Growth includes working through self-limiting thoughts, habits, and behaviors to make positive changes in your life and progress forward.

Spirituality is based on your own personal definition of the term, but it may include religion (if practiced) and connection — the feeling that you're part of something greater than yourself.

Family and Friends includes relationships outside of that with your significant other.

Romance includes your relationship with your significant other/intimate partner.

Recreation includes fun, hobbies, and creative expression.

Environment includes your home, the physical location of your home, and pets.

Once you complete your wheel of life, you'll move onto completing the following questions. For these questions, you can either write your responses on the printed worksheet, or you can write them in your journal. These questions will allow you to examine what you want for each area to increase your level of satisfaction in life.

As you look at each area of your life, ask yourself how you'll know when you've reached a level 10 in each area. Describe the ideal conditions for each area of your life. Don't think in terms of what you think is or is not possible.

Thought questions are provided for each area, but please don't feel limited by them. They're just there to get you to start thinking about what you want for each area.

Career: Are you in your ideal job? If not, what is your ideal job? Do you want to start a business? Do you want to go back to school? Do you want to write a book? How will you know when you have your ideal career?

Finances: Are you happy with your financial situation? If not, what would it take to get there? How much do you want in your savings, investments, and retirement? How much do you want to make per year? Do you want to be out of debt?

Contribution: How do you want to serve your community and the world at large? What causes are important to you? How much money and time do you want to give to these causes?

Health: How will you know when you've achieved your ideal level of health? How will you feel? What vision do you have for your physical body? What about your emotional health and overall wellbeing?

Personal Growth: What do you want to do to grow personally? How many books do you want to read per month? What trainings do you want to attend? Do you want to work with a mentor or coach? Do you have habits and behaviors that no longer serve you in a positive way that you want to replace?

Spirituality: What does spirituality mean to you? Does it include religion? Do you feel that you're part of something greater than yourself? How much time do you want to spend in meditation or prayer each day?

Family and Friends: What is your ideal relationship with your family and friends? Do you wish you had a better relationship with specific family members? Do you wish you had more friends? Are there some people in your life that you need to distance yourself from?

Romance: What is your ideal relationship with your current partner? If you are seeking a relationship, what are you looking for in an intimate relationship?

Recreation: What brings you the most enjoyment? What do you do that excites you? What activities make you smile? What are some activities you've always wanted to try?

Environment: Are you happy in your home and work environment? What kind of home would you love to live in? How would it be decorated? Where would it be located?

This activity isn't meant to make you feel bad for where you currently are in your life. It's also not about saying you must work on a specific area just because there's a gap. It's simply an awareness-building activity. Before you set goals for moving forward, it's helpful to first have a good understanding of where you currently are. This way, you can also consider whether the goal you want to pursue is the right one to pursue at this time or whether pursuing another goal might be more useful to you. Later on, I'll discuss why it's important to focus on one goal at a time so you don't get overwhelmed. The wheel of life is an effective tool to use when deciding which goal to set your sights on first.

Outcome Specification

Once you identify the gap between where you are now and where you want to be, it's time to set goals to begin to decrease that gap. As a Certified Neuro-Linguistic Programming (NLP) Practitioner, I find the outcome specification model, an NLP technique for setting goals, very useful. I find the process so useful that I included it as an integral component of The BOSS Technique, a coaching method I created to help my clients move forward from their unchangeable past. The O in BOSS stands for outcome specification.

As the name implies, outcome specification is about getting very specific about the goal—the outcome—you're looking to achieve. As Tom Hopkins said in *The Official Guide to Success*, "Undefined goals are unreachable."[6] The outcome specification process can be used for any type of goal, big or small. It allows you to look at the goal you want to achieve, drill down to the nitty-gritty details on why you want to achieve the goal, and create a plan for how you're going to achieve it.

Part of why trauma can be so devastating is because it signifies a loss of control. Setting goals and a plan of action to achieve those goals, is extremely empowering and is an important step in taking back control of your life. Throughout a sequence of activities in the remainder of this chapter, you'll be examining in detail one specific goal you would like to achieve that will make the biggest difference in your life when you achieve it. You can always examine other goals later, but for this activity, you'll need to pick *one* to work on. Pursuing multiple goals at once will be very overwhelming, and you'll likely achieve few, if any, of the goals because you'll be more likely to give up.

You may not want to write certain goals down because you don't even know where to begin, but try not to worry about the "how" just yet. The how will be examined at a later point. In the meantime, it may be helpful to keep in mind that the universe is quite amazing. As Paulo Coelho stated in his book, *The Alchemist*, "When you want something, all the universe conspires in helping you to achieve it."[7] I've found this to be true in my own life. When I start working toward a goal, the people and resources I need to achieve that goal just seem to appear in my path. However, it doesn't work like magic. It happens because I'm hyperfocused on the goal I'm aiming for, and all the actions I take are to drive me toward that one goal. Taking the necessary steps to achieve a desired goal will guide you along the path that will include all the resources you need.

Chapter 5 will be dedicated to taking action on your goals. This is where the "how" of your goal will come to fruition. Right now, just focus on naming the goal. I recommend you get out your Wheel of Life worksheet from the last activity. Looking at your goals and your wheel, choose one area of your life that would have the greatest influence on all the others if you were to improve that one area. Then pick one goal in that area of your life to begin working on.

I'm hopeful that by examining your wheel and reading the coming paragraphs, you'll be able to decide which area of your life to focus on first. However, if you get to the point of writing down a goal and you still have no idea what to write, pick a goal in the health category to start working on. This category is particularly powerful because when you feel better, you'll have the energy to tackle other aspects of your life. Then pick one specific facet of your health to work on first, such as your sleep, exercise, diet, or emotional health. You can't go wrong with any of these categories, so pick one and use it to progress through the next activity. You can always change your goal later, but it's important to have a goal to start with.

When determining the goal you want to work on, it's important to examine it and determine if it's really what *you* want. You should ask yourself: "Is someone else or society dictating what my goals should be?" When my students weren't doing well in class and I knew that they weren't committing the time necessary to be successful, I would ask them if they still wanted to do the degree program and why they chose it in the first place. I often got answers like, "My parents told me I had to get a job or go to school, so I chose school", "I wanted to study art, but my friends and family told me that wasn't realistic, and to get into healthcare where I could always find a job", or "My employer is requiring that I complete a higher degree or I'll lose my job".

It's so common for people to strive for a career, a body, home, car, and vacations that others think are acceptable but may not necessarily be what they want. It's unlikely that you'll ever be truly happy on a path of someone else's choosing. It's time to start deciding what you want out of your life and not let everyone else's priorities take over your own.

I also recognize that writing down your goals might be challenging because you don't know what's possible or don't believe that the goals you want to achieve are possible. Limiting beliefs will be discussed further in Chapter 4, but I think this is a very important time to start recognizing what self-limiting beliefs you might have. If you want to write a goal down but you stop yourself because a voice in your head says that it's not possible, you're crazy, or a voice from someone in your past or present life is telling you that what you want to achieve isn't possible, still write it down. Then we'll address those limiting beliefs in Chapter 4.

I encourage you to listen to motivational audio that will inspire you and hopefully show you what's possible for you and your life. If you go to my website at serotinouslife.com/help you can sign up to receive access to a list of my favorite books, videos, and articles on healing from trauma and coping with life's daily stressors. In the videos sections, you'll see a link for "Motivation and Inspiration". This will bring you to a YouTube playlist of some of my favorite motivational and inspirational speakers, many of which have overcome great hardship. These stories of overcoming hardship and showing what's possible are important. People have difficulty striving for goals they don't think are possible. These kinds of speeches provide hope and clarity about what's truly possible.

Listening to audiobooks, YouTube videos, and podcasts helped change the destructive narrative that I had set on repeat in my mind. From years of trauma, I developed numerous limiting beliefs that got in the way of me living the life I desired and deserved. Having mentors like the business philosopher, Jim Rohn, helped me pivot when I was off track. Keep in mind that I never met Jim Rohn and never will, as he passed away, but he continues to provide guidance through his books and videos.

I have many mentors that I've never met and I encourage you to do the same. You don't have to meet someone in person for them to influence your life. That's the power of books, audio, and video recordings. A person can be long gone and you can still learn from their message. Or, perhaps they're still alive, but maybe you'll never have the opportunity to meet them. Through the evergreen resources they've created, you can still learn from them and grow from what you learn.

Although some goals may take years to achieve, we can stay on track by keeping the words of our mentors flowing into our mind. Or they can help you right yourself when you get off track. Mentors are invaluable.

As you're moving through the activities in the remainder of this chapter, it's important to acknowledge why you want to pursue a goal that could knock so many other areas out of balance, if that's the case. If your career already causes your health and relationships to suffer, it's important to examine why you want to pursue an even bigger career goal. What are you really trying to achieve, and could it be achieved in another way that wouldn't cause so much stress in other areas of your life? Or do you have certain limiting beliefs or insecurities that need to be addressed? Please consider these things as you move through the next activities.

You want to choose goals that will improve multiple areas of your life. Oftentimes people choose goals like financial goals or career goals that actually deplete other areas of their lives like their health or relationships. Then they spend their lives with regrets about the time they didn't spend with their children or the time they didn't spend with their family and friends that are no longer around. They skimp on sleep and eat like crap while they're working multiple hours a day, and they're not exercising. Then they end up spending all sorts of time and money trying to get their health back later on in life, likely when it's too late.

That's also why you want to make sure that your goals are in line with your values. If all the goals you choose in life are in line with your values, then you're going to have a life filled with meaningful experiences. That way, even if you don't achieve your goals, you'll have lived a meaningful life and one that you can be proud of. If you value time with your family, then you should take this into consideration when setting goals that could cause you to have less time with your family. However, this doesn't mean that you can't work on building a business while you have a job just because it'll cause you to spend less time with your family.

Maybe you want to pursue the business because you see it as a way to have more time with the ones you love. In this case, I recommend that you have a sit-down discussion with your loved ones and explain why you want to achieve this goal, the short-term effects it'll have on the family dynamic, and the benefits achieving this goal could bring to the family in the future. This will give your family the opportunity to voice their concerns. When their concerns are heard and recognized as valid, then you can brainstorm ways that the family connection can remain strong while you're pursuing your goal. Maybe the family can be involved in different facets of the process. This way, you're maintaining connections with your family and progressing toward your goal at the same time.

It's very likely that as you read through this book, you'll want to change the original goal you chose because you might not think the same way by the end of this book as you did at the beginning. Just start by choosing a goal to work on based on where you are right now. It's no big deal if you come back and change it in a few hours, days, or weeks from now.

Activity: Identify the Specific Goal You Want to Achieve

It'll be easiest to complete this activity and the remaining activities in this chapter if you print out the Outcome Specification worksheet. You can access this worksheet at serotinouslife.com/worksheets. However, if you don't currently have access to a printer, you can use your journal to record your responses.

Pick one goal that would make the biggest difference in your life if you were to achieve it. It's difficult for us to stay intensely focused on too many goals at once. So, choose the one goal that means the most to you. It doesn't have to be an enormous goal to start out. Meet yourself where you currently are. Don't try to push yourself farther and faster than you're ready to go, or you'll likely get discouraged and give up on your goal.

When you're writing your goal, make sure it meets each of the following requirements:

- State your goal in positive terms, meaning what you do want (positive), not what you don't want (negative).
- Be self-directed. Your goal should be within your control. It shouldn't be based on another person doing or not doing something. Don't put your future in someone else's hands.

- Choose an appropriately sized goal. Have you ever achieved or come close to achieving a goal like this in the past? Is your goal too much for you to cope with? Will you be motivated right through to completion? If it's a big goal, set a smaller goal that will lead you to achieving the bigger goal.
- When, where, and with whom do you want to achieve it?

Designing our future can be so exciting. It can help us feel a sense of control over our lives. It can give us hope that tomorrow will be even better than today. That's why I hope you'll take the time to sit down and really think about your goals and what you want for your life. Even though it might not always seem like it at the time, you have the ability to change how you're experiencing life at any moment you choose. Change doesn't always require a big pivot in your life. Sometimes it's just about shifting your mindset so you think differently about your life circumstances. Shifting your perspective will be a primary focus of Chapter 4.

For now, just start by making a commitment to yourself by writing one goal down. That's it. Just one. Regardless of how big or small it is, it's an important first step in changing how you're experiencing life.

What is Your Why?

Why did you decide to read this book? Why did you choose the goal you did in the previous activity? We're often oblivious to the factors that drive our behaviors and goals. We say we want a million dollars without really understanding why we want that. What we don't realize is, often it isn't the money we're looking for, it's the sense of security or accomplishment that's associated with that amount of money. We say we want to lose 10 pounds without really understanding what the real reason is behind that goal. We might say that it's to feel better and look better, but maybe the real reason is that we feel concerned that our significant other will cheat on us or leave us if we don't lose the weight.

In the next activity, you'll identify why doing this work is important to you. This will help to keep you motivated when things are difficult. It'll allow you to identify your pain points. What pain are you currently suffering, and what beauty are you missing out on by not moving past your trauma?

One technique you'll be using in the next activity is the *5 Whys* technique. It's called the *5 Whys* because, on average, it takes asking why 5 times before you get down to the real reason you want to achieve a specific goal. However, don't hesitate to ask why 6, 7, or more times if you feel you haven't dug deep enough yet. You'll likely find that the first *why* you start out with is much different than the fifth. Your fifth *why* is usually the real, deep, and truly meaningful reason behind why you want to make a change. You begin to realize that your true motivation for wanting to achieve a specific goal is much bigger than what you initially realized. Becoming aware of your real motivation will fuel you to keep moving forward.

The next activity will help reveal your real motivation for reading this book. Through this and the remaining activities in this chapter, you'll have the opportunity to examine what will stay the same if you don't achieve the transformation you're looking for and how your life will be different once you do achieve it.

When you first ask yourself why you want to achieve the goal you're aiming for, you'll find that your first *why* tends to be superficial. By the time you get down to your fifth *why*, you're getting into the deep-rooted reasons behind why you want to achieve this goal. You'll see this with an example from my own life in the next activity.

My goal was to lose weight, so I started out with saying I wanted to lose weight so I could feel better. And this is where most people stop without questioning themselves further. When I got right down to it, my reason for losing weight was actually tied to my full-time job. By doing this exercise yourself, you'll begin to see that your goal is typically much bigger than you originally realized. You'll likely even begin to see how your goal is related to other aspects of your wheel of life. I started out wanting to improve the health category in my life, but in reality, by improving the health category, I would also improve my career category and ultimately many of the other categories as well.

If you're not wanting to complete the work in the next exercise, or at any point in this book, I encourage you to journal about why that is. Are you afraid that you won't be able to handle the difficult emotions that come up? If that's the case, I encourage you to develop a self-care plan to handle those emotions so they don't overwhelm you. There are so many things that you can do if you start flooding with emotion. Some options are to sit back, close your eyes, and take a few deep breaths; go for a walk; or call a friend. In the future, when the going gets tough, you'll need your 5 *Whys* to remind yourself why this work is important to you.

Activity: 5 Whys

Complete the 5 *Whys* exercise for the reason you want to achieve the one goal you identified in the previous activity. Ask yourself why you want to achieve this goal at least 5 times to get down to the real reason behind why it's important to you. Each answer forms the basis of the next question. Here's an example from my own life. My goal is to get my weight down to 135 pounds.

Why do you want to lose weight? So I can feel better (first why).

Why do you want to feel better? So I won't feel so tired throughout the day (second why).

Why don't you want to feel tired throughout the day? So I can get more accomplished (third why).

Why do you want to get more accomplished? So my business will grow quicker (fourth why).

Why do you want your business to grow quicker? So I can leave my soul-sucking job (fifth why).

Now it's your turn. Take out your Outcome Specification worksheet or journal and ask yourself why you want to achieve the goal you chose in the last activity at least 5 times, to get down to the real reason you want to achieve the goal.

It might be helpful to put your *why* on a note card or sticky note, and place it where it can easily be seen so you can regularly be reminded of why this goal is important to you. We're often encouraged to put everyone's needs above our own, for our family, career, or community. It'll be easy to fall off track after you start moving toward your goals if you continue to let everyone else's priorities take over your own.

Having a quick reminder to yourself of why you should make yourself your top priority in your life will be helpful in preventing you from falling back into old patterns. Or, it'll at least help you to get back on track when you do get temporarily sidelined.

Digging Down Deep

The next activity will have you evaluate multiple facets of achieving your goal. You'll have the opportunity to examine what your life would be like if you don't reach your goal. You'll determine how you'll know when you've achieved your goal. You'll be asked why you haven't pursued this goal before now, or if you have, why you stopped moving forward in the past. You'll explore the resources you already have and any additional resources you'll need to achieve your goal. You'll also be examining how the pursuit of your goal might affect the important people in your life and what you might have to give up or sacrifice to reach this goal. This is another chance to examine your wheel of life and see if this goal will knock certain parts out of balance. That is expected at times.

If you have a child, especially when the baby is first born, it's very likely that other areas of your life will be affected. If you're going back to school or starting a business, other areas might also be affected, but this is also your opportunity to determine if those costs are worth it. Many times they will be, but sometimes they might not. This is where it's of particular importance to talk about your goals with the people closest to you in your life that could be affected by the pursuit of your goal. When it's all said and done, you might decide not to pursue your goal, and that's okay, but you want to make sure that whether you pursue your goal or not, it's your decision and you're happy with the choices you've made.

For example, if your goal is to lose 20 pounds, how will that affect your partner and family if you'll no longer be going out to eat with them, or cooking the same meals, or deserts? Will your partner start to become self-conscious? You might need to reassure your partner that you aren't looking to attract anyone else into your life. They might be concerned of you cheating on them or that you'll leave them once you do lose weight.

Depending on how you choose to lose weight, it might affect the time you're at home or your meals together. If you start going to the gym for one hour per day, three days per week, that's less time you'll have to spend with your family. So you need to make sure they understand why you're doing this and it might take continual reminders. If you start eating differently, they might not want to do the same. Then you have to determine how you'll handle that. Will you eat entirely different meals together, or will you make it an adventure and have the whole family try new foods? None of these questions are meant to deter you from pursuing your goal. They're so you can go into your goal with your eyes wide open so you can anticipate issues you may encounter while in pursuit of your goal.

If you want to stop drinking or smoking, how would that affect those around you? Did you use to have time to have conversations with family and friends while you were smoking, and now they won't have that time with you any longer? Again, this is not to say that you have to give up your goal if it'll make someone else uncomfortable, it's just for you to be aware that pursuing your goal might affect those around you. If you don't take these things into consideration ahead of time, they might appear as obstacles in your path while pursuing your goal. You want to try your best to make those around you feel safe and secure so they can feel comfortable supporting you in meeting your goals.

The next activity will ask you to evaluate the daily actions you'll need to take to achieve your goal and immediate actions you can begin to take. This topic will be revisited in Chapter 5, which will cover breaking your goal down into bite-sized pieces and taking action. But right now, I want you to think about whether this goal is worth it to you. To really determine that, you must have an idea of what actions you're going to need to take to achieve that goal and whether you're even interested in doing what's necessary to reach that goal.

Activity: Digging Down Deep

Get out your Outcome Specification worksheet or journal and answer each of the following questions:
- What's going to happen if you don't reach your goal? What's not going to happen if you don't reach your goal?

- How will you know when you've reached your goal? What will be your evidence of success? What will the outcome look like, sound like, and feel like? Sit back and immerse yourself in all the sensations you would feel when you achieve your goal.
- Where, or in what situation(s) will the goal be relevant? Where might it be irrelevant? For example, if you have a goal to be more adventurous, in what situations might being adventurous be safe or appropriate and in what situations would it not be?
- Why haven't you started pursuing this goal before now? If you have, what has stopped you from pursuing this goal wholeheartedly?
- What resources do you already possess that you can draw upon to help you achieve your goal (e.g., determination, specific skills)?
- What additional personal resources will you need to achieve your goal (e.g., patience, perseverance)?
- How might the pursuit of your goal affect the important people in your life? Is there anything that you would have to give up or sacrifice to reach this goal?
- What are the daily actions you'll need to take to achieve your goal? What's the first step you can take today?
- Given everything you've considered to this point, is achieving this goal worth the effort and sacrifice? Why?

It's completely okay if after going through this process, you decide the initial goal you chose is not what you want to pursue. I encourage you to reflect on why you now don't want to achieve that goal. Is it because you think it'll be too hard? Is it because you're scared? If it turns out that the fear of failure or the fear of what people will think, is what's holding you back, then I encourage you to see if you want to reevaluate giving up after you've considered everything in the coming chapters. You might end up deciding to move forward even though you're scared and it'll be hard.

The next chapter will discuss ego. If you only want to achieve your goal because of ego, instead of it actually bringing fulfillment to your life, the next chapter might cause you to rethink your goal. And that's okay. It's okay to set a goal and change your mind. It's your life, and you deserve to experience life in the way you choose. If you choose one path and it turns out to not be the direction you want to move in, you always have the option to pivot. You can make slight alterations or a complete overhaul of your goals at any point.

I encourage you to come back to this chapter once you finish the book to determine if you want to stay committed to the initial goal you chose. I also encourage you to come back to this chapter when you're ready to pursue new goals in the future. Finally, I encourage you to save the Outcome Specification worksheet to your computer so you can always access it and print it out each time you want to set a new goal. You can do the same with the Wheel of Life worksheet so you can have a visual of how a new goal may affect multiple aspects of your life.

Chapter 3
What Will People Think?

Many people resist setting big goals because they're worried about failing and falling flat on their faces. They worry about other people saying, "I told you so. I knew you couldn't do it." This desire to get approval from others holds people back all the time and keeps them stagnating in a life that they don't even want because they're afraid of what other people are going to think if they fail. What people fail to realize is that most people don't want to see you achieving more than they've achieved themselves. They want to keep you down because it makes them feel better about themselves, so much so that when you start climbing higher, they might actively try to bring you down.

A lot of this isn't even conscious. They do it subconsciously without even thinking. The moment you start climbing higher, it's going to put a mirror up to them. This mirror is going to force them to look at themselves in the face and see what they're not doing to change their life circumstances. By keeping you small, they're going to feel bigger and better about themselves. This is why you must be careful of who you're giving away your power and your future to. You must always ask yourself: does this person have my best interest in mind? Unfortunately, the answer will often be "no". It doesn't necessarily mean they're a bad person, it's just that if they're floundering in their own life and struggling to take care of their own needs, how on Earth will they be able to make sure that your needs are taken care of too? They answer is, they can't. Instead, their natural instinct will be to bring you back down as you're climbing so it doesn't make them feel bad about where they are at in their own life.

We are deeply social creatures. From an evolutionary standpoint, it makes perfect sense why we care what people think. If we do something that other people perceive as strange or out of the norm, we might be ostracized. Historically, being excluded from the group could mean a threat to our survival. Given our natural instinct to want to remain as part of a group, it's no wonder why most people are scared of public speaking, standing up for someone that's being put down by their group, and pursuing a goal that no one in the group has ever achieved before. All could result in them being excluded from the group. Even though this is instinctual, it can be overridden. Yes, it can be scary, but it can be done.

As children, it can be difficult to go against your group because your survival still largely depends on your parents. If your parents never encouraged you to be vulnerable, push your limits, and do things even though you were scared, it makes doing these things as adults even scarier because you never had practice. But that doesn't mean you can't practice once you leave the nest.

Although growing up in a small town has its benefits, it has its definite drawbacks. In the town I grew up in Upstate, New York, my friend's parents and my parents went to school together, and our grandparents went to school together. Many people never leave, and if they do, they rarely come back, so you get a collection of people who think very similarly. Most of our teachers also grew up in and around our town. With few new people moving into our town, new ideas and new ways of thinking were rarely introduced. This means that if you did something out of the norm, you were often criticized by all levels of the community. This is why it took pure grit and determination to not allow my way of thinking to be warped by their resistance to change. That's why I had to get out.

Most of my traumas occurred in the town I grew up in. Secrets were kept because it's a small town. Victimizers weren't brought to justice because it's a small town. Abuses perpetuate from one generation to the next because secrets must be kept in a small town because, once one person knows, everyone knows. So why will you tell when you're victimized again and again by other people when you know that nothing will happen because it's a small town? You don't.

Many people from my hometown were shocked when they heard that I was sexually violated by eight different men in and around our small town, from the ages of 9 to 19. They never knew because I kept all but one abuse to myself because of who my victimizers were and how they shamed me so I would be too embarrassed to tell, and because I knew that nothing would be done after the bad experiences I had telling.

What I experienced in my hometown isn't unique to my hometown. It's common in all small towns and small communities within big cities. People don't share their secrets because they're afraid of getting ostracized from the group. The family members of the victimizers are at threat of being ostracized. The family members of the victim are threatened with being ostracized as well. Victims are threatened with being deemed an outcast because people often look at you with pity or as being unclean after being sexually violated. If you're a parent, people look at you with contempt and condemnation for not protecting your child. It's about self-preservation.

From my years teaching about evolution, I now understand this desire to not be excluded from the group. However, as a child, I operated based on my instincts. My instincts told me that carrying the weight of my trauma in silence was not only for my own good but the good of my whole family. It's why I still won't publicly name my victimizers. I know some people don't understand that, but it's still ingrained in me to think about how sharing secrets will ripple throughout my family and community.

I want to be clear that I'm not trying to denigrate the town I grew up in. I still have many family members and friends that live there and I don't want to condemn the community. Yes, terrible things happened to me there. Yes, faulty ways of thinking perpetuate cycles of abuse. But again, what I experienced in my hometown is not unique to my hometown. These are issues that can be found throughout rural communities or small, close-knit communities within larger communities when you're not interacting with people other than those in your tight circle.

In small communities, people often think the same. If there are no new people regularly moving into the community, or if people leave and never come back, then new ways of thinking are never introduced into the community. So people become very close minded. That's why I think it's important that any young person who grows up in a small town or in a close-knit community where they don't have exposure to people outside of their own culture, actively seek out ways to gain exposure to new ways of thinking. You can do this by going to college where you'll have the opportunity to meet people from different places. You can also do it through different kinds of learning experiences such as volunteering locally or internationally.

If you're in a small community and you currently don't have the means for getting out, or you're too young to leave your parents' household, you can access alternate ways of thinking through books, videos on YouTube, and podcasts. You can read and listen to people with different opinions to expand your horizons of what's possible.

Now that I'm an adult, I realize that everyone in my hometown, my family, friends, teachers, and neighbors were all doing the very best they could. But that doesn't mean that things couldn't have been handled differently. It doesn't mean that it's okay for abuses to continue in small communities and for adults not to do anything about it, or for victims to stay silent. It means that I don't look at the town and the people in it as terrible, however I must acknowledge that there's a specific culture that requires you to act in a certain way to fit in. It means that it's hard to go against the grain and pursue a goal that seems absurd to family and friends that think it isn't possible. It means that I had the perfect training ground to develop a deep sense of grit, determination, and perseverance to go against the pack and eventually leave the pack. It was difficult but it provided me proof that, not only could I go against my social group and survive, but

I could also leave my social group altogether and thrive on my own.

Unfortunately, our brains don't realize that we're no longer in danger of saber-toothed tigers lurking around the corner if we're laughed away from our group. Our brain still responds with the same flood of fight-or-flight chemicals when we're nervous about walking out on stage, leaving a full-time job to start a business, or standing up for the rights of someone that our group has chosen to exclude. Due to the release of the same chemicals, we can experience the same level of fear as if we were truly in danger of being eaten by a saber-toothed tiger.

The bottom line is that you need to practice going against the grain and seeing that you'll be okay if the group doesn't accept you. As the late author, Dr. Susan Jeffers would say, "Feel the fear and do it anyway." It takes going up on stage and seeing that, even after everyone laughed at you, you still survived. It takes writing that book and seeing that, even though it didn't get published, even though your loved ones told you that your idea was crazy, you still survived. It takes leaving that teaching job for a sales job to reach your financial goals, and seeing that you survived even though everyone made fun of you. Once you know that you can do something scary (something that the group doesn't agree with) and survive, you'll be more likely to push out the boundaries of your comfort zone a little farther.

I'm constantly doing this. I do this with my traveling, mountain adventures, and career. The more times I prove to myself that I can step outside of my comfort zone when I'm scared and still survive, the bigger chance I'm willing to take in the future. My life keeps getting better and better each year that I'm alive

Be Kind to Yourself

As liberating as reframing and setting goals for the future can be, it's not always going to be easy. It's going to take constant work to not slip into your old patterns of thinking and behaving. So, please be patient and kind to yourself along the way. Expect that you're going to slip up. Even if you start off doing really great with new habits and working toward the goals you've set for yourself, something will definitely trigger you along the way. There will be people or circumstances that cause you to want to take a step back. It's during these times that you must show yourself love and compassion.

You must remember that these old patterns have been ingrained in you for years, so it's going to take time to break them. You're going to engage in old patterns, or at least you're going to want to. That's why writing down your goals and regularly coming back and reflecting on them is important. It'll keep you in touch with your *why*, it'll let you know when you're off track, and it'll nudge you back on to the proper course to reach your goal.

Remember that every habit, belief, and behavior you have has served you in some way, and maybe they're excuses for you to not make a change. Change is hard; it requires you to leave your comfort zone and leave the existence that you've known for a significant portion of your life. We want to stay comfortable. Even if a habit, belief, or behavior is harming us in some way, it's still a safe space for us. It's still what we know. It's why we keep harmful habits and harmful people in our lives—it's easy. It's a known quantity.

Leaving the known for the unknown is uncomfortable and scary. Your mind will naturally wonder if the next situation you're heading toward will be worse than where you currently are, so be ready for resistance. No matter if you're currently experiencing pain from life that fear over the unknown will keep drawing you back to the comfort of your old patterns or people that may be toxic to you.

Expect that you'll get off track from time to time, but remember each day is a new beginning. When you start to get off track from any of your goals or commitments, know that it's part of the journey. Just come back to your goal—your point of focus—the next day, and if you need to apologize to yourself or others, do it, but don't wallow in regret. This is why I love meditation so much, and why I dedicated my largest chapter to it in my first book, *Transformation After Trauma*.

Meditation trains you to keep coming back to your point of focus each time you get off track. That's why it's called a practice. People often don't practice meditation because they think they're not good at it, because they get distracted so easily. But the point of meditation is to practice coming back to your point of focus each time you get off track. Over time, it'll get easier to pull yourself back to your point of focus. However, be ready to pull yourself back again and again. In the same way, be ready to recommit yourself to your goals and to yourself over and over. Know that you're worth every bit of energy and time it'll take for you to break old patterns so you can move into the life you desire and deserve.

Chapter 5
Taking Action

I've found that most people resist setting goals because they worry about what people will think, or they allow the negative chitter-chatter in their head to start eating away at their aspirations. That's why I took what might have appeared to be a detour from the goal setting process to discuss soul-suckers, ego, bad habits, and limiting beliefs. It's essential to examine these factors because they're the likely culprits behind why you haven't moved forward toward your goals already, or why you started and stopped along the way.

Now that you've examined how you and other people may be preventing you from progressing toward your goals, it's time to continue with the goal setting process. The reason I asked you to write down your goal and thoughts surrounding it, is because writing down your goals makes them real. As the writer Michael Korda says, "Write it down. Written goals have a way of transforming wishes into wants; cant's into cans; dreams into plans; and plans into reality. Don't just think it - ink it!"

Writing down your goals is a way to make a commitment to yourself. Unfortunately, many people avoid writing down their goals because then it'll either force them to take action or it'll make them feel bad for not taking action when they later look at their written goal. However, if you want to change the way you're experiencing life, you must actively work to make change happen. As we know, nothing changes if nothing changes. This is why I had you examine what has made you say "Enough is enough" and identify the real reason you want to achieve your set goal. This is so you can push through the discomfort you'll inevitably face on the way to making any change in your life. You deserve the opportunity to experience life in new ways and you're worth the time and energy it'll require to experience this change.

I use Google Docs and Sheets to keep track of my goals and progress. That way I can edit the documents from my phone or computer and always have access to them. I have one Google Doc that I titled "My Goals". I use this document to keep track of my overarching goals for all different aspects of my life. Don't stress out about working on multiple different aspects of your life right now. Stay focused on the one goal that you've chosen to work on first. I just want you to know how I keep track of multiple goals in my life.

You can tackle other goals simultaneously by having regular routines set around your main goal so they become easy. Once working toward your main goal becomes automatic, progressing toward additional goals won't be difficult. You just don't want to set additional goals early on, because working on too many goals at once before you have habits created will get you overwhelmed, and you won't likely succeed at any of them. Focus on your main goal first, and later you can reach for goals in multiple aspects of your life.

In the "My Goals" document, I like to break my goals down by year. So I list the year and then I use bullets underneath each year to indicate my major goals for that year. I include things like trainings I'd like to participate in, adventures I'd like to have, and financial goals I want to reach. Once I complete each goal, I use strikethrough to indicate that it's been completed. And if I wasn't able to complete a specific goal, I just cut and paste it to another year. I also use this document to write down thoughts around each goal, for example my motivation for wanting to achieve a specific goal, why I set the chosen deadline, and obstacles I may face along the way.

I have another Google Doc titled "Daily Goals". It's really what I use as my calendar to keep track of my appointments and specific deadlines, but I like to think of everything in the document as progress toward bigger goals. I'll talk more about how I use this document in the Routines section of this chapter because it helps minimize the number of decisions I must make and how much I need to pull from my memory each day.

I also use a Google Sheet to track my daily activities that I do to get me closer to my larger goals. I titled it "Daily Activities". I use it to make note of whether or not I complete certain activities each day, such as my meditation, stretching, and water intake. I use it as my personal accountability system, which is why I'll bring it up again at the end of this chapter when I discuss accountability.

Another helpful tip is to create a vision board. You can put it in a location where you'll always be able to see it so you have a consistent reminder of what you want to achieve. I find it helps me stay the course when things get hard. It gives me a visual reminder of my target and my *why* for aiming for it. It might be helpful to put a ladder or staircase on your vision board and write out the different mini-goals that lead up to the big goal. Having them there will remind you that, even though your goal may seem far away, each little win you achieve is getting you one step closer to it.

Getting Started

Writing down your goals is not enough, you must take action. Taking action particularly in the beginning can feel *so* hard, and that's why I love the book, *The Compound Effect* by Darren Hardy. It reinforces the importance of breaking down your goals into small manageable steps so that you'll not only be more likely to take action, but you'll also be more likely to keep making progress because you won't get overwhelmed.

If you choose a long-term goal that might take many years to achieve, you'll need to chunk it down into manageable bite-sized pieces. If your goal is too large and too overwhelming, you'll be more likely to give up. So create a plan to start taking small steps each day toward achieving your bigger end goal.

When writing this book, I would have gotten overwhelmed if I focused on the immensity of the project. So, to avoid this, I committed to working on this book for one hour every morning. I didn't set a target number of words or pages to complete, I simply committed to working on this book for one hour per day. I decided that whatever I achieve in that one hour would be good enough. Obviously, chunking down the book this way totally worked! This book is a product of simple daily disciplines that compounded into significant results over time.

If you have a weight loss goal, think of one small change you can start to make with either your diet or physical activity. You could swap out one cup of soda with one cup of water. You could even use carbonated water if you like the sensation of soda in your mouth. Even if you drink multiple cups of soda a day, still start with swapping just one cup. Once you have that down, swap out two, and so on until you're no longer drinking soda.

If you choose to start with your physical activity, begin with just progressing a little beyond what you're currently doing. If you're not currently exercising at all, start with incorporating a 5-minute walk each day, then move it to 10 minutes until you progress up to 30 minutes each day. If 30 minutes is too much at one time, you can spread it out so you do three 10-minute walks or two 15-minute walks each day. The point is, you want to start with steps that won't overwhelm you, steps that are easily achievable considering where you currently are. Over time, you can gradually increase your efforts and push yourself just a little harder until you achieve your goal. These small efforts will build like a snowball and compound into significant results over time.

Although I've hiked hundreds of mountains since 2012 when I began hiking, I didn't start with doing the largest first. I started hiking when I was morbidly obese, so every little hill felt as big as Mount Everest. I started with doing local trails that were mostly flat, then I progressed into local mountains. After that, I moved into the tallest mountains in the surrounding New York State parks. The point is, I started with hikes with the shortest distances first. As time went on, I began hiking taller peaks with more distance and started hiking more than one mountain in a day.

Eventually, I was hiking over 100 mountains per year and traveling around the United States and the world.

I like doing difficult hikes for the physical and mental challenge of it. I feel that the mountains are a perfect training ground for life. It can be difficult to hike for 12 or 13 hours in one day when my feet, knees, and back hurt. When the going gets tough, I can't afford to focus on the remaining miles I have to cover or the change in elevation, or I'll get overwhelmed. Instead, I remind myself to focus on the one step in front of me because I can always take one more step. This is how I chunk down my hiking into bite-sized pieces. If you focus on the immensity of your goal—the literal or figurative mountain you're trying to climb—it'll seem insurmountable. However, if you break down the space between where you are now and where you want to be into manageable parts, it'll be easier to close the gap.

It's important to prioritize your health, no matter your goal. What I've found is, most people pursue their goals to the detriment of their health. They skimp on sleep and exercise and spend less time on grocery shopping and meal prep. However, that's not the way to go. It's difficult to maintain focus and have the energy to commit to the different facets of your life if you don't feel well. Therefore, as you pursue your goal, it's essential to nourish your body with healthy foods, exercise, and sleep. It's also essential to nourish your mind with positive inputs that won't sap your energy but will give you the motivation to keep moving forward even when it's tough.

When you begin working toward a new goal, it's important to identify the things you spend time on, or the things you could be doing each day to get you closer to your goal. It's also important to evaluate the activities that could be sabotaging your efforts. It could be that some of your current habits aren't in line with your goal. Ask yourself: Do I need to spend as much time watching TV, scrolling through social media, looking at the news, or engaging in gossip and idle chit-chat? If I'm trying to improve my financial situation, should I be splurging on new outfits and accessories? Should I be going out to eat as often? When you do go out to eat, evaluate what adjustments you could make. For example, you could replace a soda or cocktail with water, and you could choose a satisfying meal rather than adding on dessert. This way you can take care of both your physical and financial health.

It's also important to evaluate the people you spend time with. Do they make you feel better about yourself? Consider your recent interactions with the individuals you spent much of your time with. Did you leave those interactions feeling more energized and better about yourself and your life, or did you leave feeling drained of positive energy and worse about yourself and your life? It's so easy to justify spending time with certain people because you think you're relaxing by spending time with them. However, if you take the time to really evaluate your interactions with them, you'll realize how much negative energy they project onto you regularly. All they do is complain about their significant other, their coworkers, and how terrible their life is. Those types of interaction can't enrich your life.

After experiencing trauma, people often gravitate toward other people who've experienced similar trauma. In some way, this is good because it can make them feel less alone in their suffering. However, bonding over one's trauma can be harmful because, many times when you're together, you'll end up talking about your trauma or complaining about how life just continues to deal you one blow after another. What I recommend is discussing not only your pain but also your recent wins with your close friends.

Most of my close friends, like myself, have been sexually violated, which explains our difficulty in building healthy relationships with food, ourselves, and others. Not only do we discuss our struggles when we're together, but we also discuss our recent wins. Our conversations allow us to connect with our day-to-day suffering and celebrate our recent success. That way we're supporting each other in both the good and bad times. I always leave these interactions feeling good. I can talk to them about things that were bothering me, and we can deliberate on the best solution. I always leave with an overall positive outlook on my life and myself. However, I have people in my life who've experienced trauma that I minimize my interactions with, even though I care about them. I understand their deep suffering, but they aren't doing the work to get out of their situation, and no matter how much I try to help them break their cycle of ruminating negative thoughts, nothing changes. They're just not ready to do the work. I can empathize with them but I can't spend much time with them because I always feel worse after the interaction, so I limit my time with them.

I encourage you to take inventory of your relationships because we dedicate a lot of our time to other people. It might even be helpful to write them down in your journal. You can write out their names and how you typically feel after you're done interacting with them. If it's hard for you to recall, then make note of how you feel the next time you interact with them. Do you feel better or worse after spending time with them? If you feel better, you should consider spending more time with them. If you feel worse, you should consider limiting your interactions with them. If you feel like they're sucking the life out of you, you should consider protecting yourself by not spending any more time with them.

As you progress toward your goal, you may have difficulty finding the time to spend with the people that enrich your life. When this happens, consider a way you can incorporate your goals in with the time you spend with them. For example, if you're trying to improve your health, ask if they want to go on a walk or bike ride with you, or if they want to go to the gym with you. If not, maybe you could get a headset and talk to them on the phone while you're walking, or talk with them on your headset while you're making dinner or cleaning up the house so you're combining activities. However, I recommend you don't talk to someone while doing an activity that requires a lot of mental focus, like reading email, text messages, or the news. You don't want the person to feel you're not listening or to constantly repeat themselves because you can't focus on what they're saying. That will start to erode away at your relationship. Activities like walking, cleaning, and cooking (unless you must read a recipe), are typically automatic and don't require a lot of mental focus. It's easier to talk with someone while doing these types of automated activities.

If you want to talk with someone you care about without combining with another activity, you could put a time limit on your conversations. I have friends and family that I can talk to for hours on the phone or each time we meet. Conversations that are engaging and enjoyable are wonderful, but if you're struggling to find time to work toward your goal, you may need to restrict the amount of time you spend with these individuals. You could tell them about your goal, activities, progress, and difficulties. Then you can explain why you need to limit the time you spend with them, even though you absolutely love spending time with them. Then you can let them know ahead of time or at the beginning of interactions how much time you can spend with them that day. Alternatively, you could have drinks, dinner or good conversations over video calls. This way you could save the time you would typically spend driving to a destination to meet with them.

Every time we say yes to one thing, we're automatically saying no to another. So what are you going to say no to in order to reach your goal? The next activity will give you the opportunity to evaluate the small steps you'll take to reach your goal and what you must say no to in order to make room for the new activities in your life. This is important because if you don't plan ahead of time, you'll soon begin to sacrifice your health. Little by little, you'll get more fatigued and multiple areas of your life will begin to suffer.

Activity

Track all your daily activities and how much time you spend on each activity. I encourage you to do this for one week, but if that overwhelms you, I encourage you to do it for a minimum of three days. Just pick three days that are most representative of the days in a typical week and make sure to pick at least one weekend day. This is an awareness building exercise.

Most of our daily activities are habits, so we usually aren't consciously aware of why we're doing certain activities or how long we spend on them. Make note of everything you do in a day, from bathing to checking email, scrolling through social media, looking at the news, watching TV, exercising, to talking to family, friends, and colleagues. This isn't the time to change anything. This is just an observational period. You want it to be an accurate representation of how you typically spend your days.

You can track your daily activities by carrying your journal or a small notebook around with you each day. You can also use a note taking app on your phone like Notes or Google Keep. This way you can make note of each activity and the duration as soon as you complete the activity. You won't be able to remember all the activities and the durations if you wait until the end of the day to record them.

If you're typically stressed out about not having enough time, I know this activity might seem overwhelming to you at first. I know you'll automatically think about how you don't have time to do this. In reality, it'll only take a few seconds to make note of each activity. Try to keep in mind how much time you'll save when you begin to take control of your days.

When people track their daily activities, they're often shocked at how much time they spend in idle chit-chat, scrolling on social media, looking at the news, or watching TV. Once you finish your tracking, look at what you spent your time on each day. It's helpful to make note of each activity on a separate page and add up the total amount spent on each activity during your tracking period. You might be shocked how much time you spend on activities that don't enrich your life.

To complete the next stage of this activity, it'll be easiest if you print out the Daily Activities worksheet. You can access this worksheet at serotinouslife.com/worksheets. However, if you don't currently have access to a printer, you can use your journal to record your responses. If you'll be using your journal, make four columns on the page. Title the first column "Keep Doing", the second column "Increase Time Spent", the third column "Decrease Time Spent", and the fourth column "Stop Doing".

To complete the chart, get out your journal, notebook, or open your mobile application with which you've been tracking your daily activities. Look at each activity and how much time you spent on each activity. When reviewing each activity, think about it in relation to your goal and the life you want to create for yourself. Ask yourself: is this activity getting me closer to or farther away from the life I desire and deserve?

If you want to keep doing a certain activity for the same amount of time, write it down in the "Keep Doing" column. If you want to keep doing the activity but you want to spend more time on it, make note of it in the "Increase Time Spent" column. Then indicate the *minimum* amount of time you want to start allocating to this activity each day. If you want to keep doing the activity but you want to spend less time on it, make note of it in the "Decrease Time Spent" column. Also, indicate the *maximum* amount of time you want to start allocating to this activity each day. For activities you want to stop doing altogether, make note of them in the "Stop Doing" column. I encourage you to print out the worksheet again or move onto another page in your journal if you run out of space.

Trading short-term comfort for a long-term gain will take discipline. Abraham Lincoln said, "Discipline is choosing between what you want now and what you want most." That means there will be discomfort in the process. You must be ready for this discomfort so you don't use it as a reason to not take action. There will be many times where you don't feel like doing the thing you need to do to move toward your goal, but you must push through and do it anyway. When I was writing this book, it took discipline to get up early and write for an hour before anything else. Most days I didn't feel like waking up early. I was tired and wanted to stay in bed, but I forced myself to get out of bed and write.

Part of my goal was to avoid checking my email, text messages, social media accounts, or the news until I finished spending one hour on writing. It took discipline to wait to do these things, particularly if I was expecting a response from someone. There were days I chose to skip writing because I was traveling or I had to get up early for a hike or podcast interview. I was comfortable doing this on these days because I'm also committed to getting adequate sleep every day and there are only so many hours in a day. I try not to sacrifice my sleep time to meet my goals because doing so can hinder my ability to focus and be creative throughout the day.

Whenever I skip a day of writing, writing the next day becomes difficult. Since I've broken my streak, I immediately start to rationalize why I could also skip the next day. I try to find an excuse for why I should stay in bed a little longer. I'm telling you this to show you how difficult changing your life can be. The road to achieving your goal will be a very bumpy one, and your strong determination will go a long way in helping you stay the course.

Every day you'll battle with the decision to choose either the short-term comfort or the long-term comfort. I know you might be scared of how tough moving forward can get, but nonetheless you'll achieve anything if you set your mind to it. Think of the trauma you've endured, yet you're still here. You survived. That's proof that you can overcome anything.

Change is uncomfortable, which is why it's difficult. Your brain looks for patterns and feels safest when your surroundings and experiences are familiar. When you start changing how you're experiencing life, your brain goes on high alert, looking around for all the things that could go wrong in an effort to keep you safe. That's why you may feel a bit of anxiety or stress when pursuing a goal because change can trigger the fight-or-flight response. Many people interpret this stress response as a warning and stop moving forward. I completely understand why they feel that way because their brain is literally telling them to be afraid of moving forward. What's interesting though is that, when people start moving forward even though they're scared, they eventually see that everything is okay. Once your brain sees that you're safe in this new situation, the stress response calms down and you can settle into this new experience. That's the main message of Dr. Susan Jeffers' book, *Feel the Fear...and Do It Anyway*. You must push through the discomfort to prove to your brain and to yourself that you can survive. You must feel the fear and do it anyway!

One technique I like to use and I think will also be helpful to you when pushing yourself to do something uncomfortable, is Mel Robbins' *5 Second Rule*. You can use the technique whenever you're hesitating taking a necessary action, whether it's speaking up for yourself, getting out of your comfortable bed, introducing yourself to someone you want to meet, or taking the first step toward a new goal. Like the spaceship countdown, you simply start counting down, "5, 4, 3, 2, 1" and then take off. Whenever I want to hit the snooze button on my alarm, I say to myself, "5, 4, 3, 2, 1" and sit up in the middle of my counting. Then I finish with saying, "Feet on the floor, Stephanie."

Additionally, I found it very useful to give myself a little extra push when it feels particularly hard. If I'm doing a final push toward a summit or getting ready to speak in front of a large group, I might say, "You got this," or "You can do hard things," just to give myself that little extra nudge of support to push me forward. Whether you give yourself extra words of encouragement at the end or not, The 5 Second Rule is great for helping you to take action when you're scared or just don't feel like taking action.

I can promise you that you will have days—many days—where you don't feel like doing the daily activities needed to progress toward your goal. That's why you must have a strategy in place to tackle days like this. You could also try pumping yourself up with upbeat music or motivational audio, but you must have a plan. I encourage you to begin trying out different strategies for forcing yourself to do the things you need to do. You know what they say: when the going gets tough, the tough get going.

Building Momentum

In the beginning of the goal setting process, you may feel extremely motivated or hopeful about making changes in your life. Designing your future can be exciting. It gives you a sense of control over your life. It gives you hope that tomorrow will be better than today. Unfortunately, excitement tends to dissipate over time and can't be depended upon to sustain momentum over the long term. That's why even though people are often excited to make a change and they go at it full steam ahead in the beginning, many will begin to peter out and end up stopping altogether. To ensure success, not only do you need to chunk down your goal into bite-sized pieces, but you also need to take the necessary daily actions toward achieving those goals to build momentum. You must take these actions whether you feel like it or not because, most days you're not going to feel like it. That's why you need to practice pushing yourself to take action when you don't feel like it. And that's why I like doing difficult hikes and setting big goals for myself; they force me to do difficult things even when I don't feel like it or when I doubt my abilities.

Building the initial momentum needed to take action can be tough. Think of an airplane during take-off. The rate of fuel consumption tends to be greater during take-off and departure than at any other time during a flight. It's not until the airplane begins a cruise climb or when it reaches cruise altitude that the fuel consumption decreases. The same is true for you. The initial momentum needed to take the actions that will push you forward toward your goal will feel the hardest. You'll need to expend the most energy and muster the most inner-strength during this period. However, once you begin to gain momentum, it won't be as difficult to keep going.

When you're moving forward toward your goal, you'll have little successes, little wins along the way that will give you encouragement to keep moving. You'll be building habits and routines that will help maintain the momentum. That's why you want to continue to maintain that momentum, because once you lose the momentum, you're going to have to rebuild it again.

If you find that you've steered off course or you've started to lose your momentum, you must bring yourself back as quickly as possible so you don't have to restart the process of rebuilding momentum again. Once that happens, it's going to feel hard like it did at the beginning. However, if you can catch yourself, you won't have to work hard on rebuilding the new habits and beliefs that are necessary to propel you toward your goal. It's also important to make sure you're moving in the right direction. As Dr. Tom Morris said in *The Seven Greatest Success Ideas*, "What good is running faster in the wrong direction?"[9]

My anxiety tends to run pretty high and gets worse when I have a lot on my plate. On September 4, 2016, my friend Sandra and I planned on hiking Mount Abraham and Mount Ellen, two of Vermont's five 4,000-foot mountains. We had almost a three-hour drive to the first trailhead. We left one car there and then drove the other car to our starting point. I did little research for this hike, which was unusual for me. I was teaching at that time, and it was the beginning of the semester. I was teaching full-time at one college and part-time at two others, so I was barely keeping my head above water. Not only did I spend little time researching the hike, but I was also more overwhelmed than usual.

When we got to the trailhead a little later than I had anticipated, I was only focusing on all the miles and elevation gain we had to cover to summit both mountains, on top of having another three-hour drive back home, so I didn't bother to check the map to make sure we were going in the right direction. I only wanted to get moving toward our goals for the day. It wasn't until over an hour after hiking that I stopped to look at the map and realized that we were heading in the wrong direction!

The trailhead we started on was on the Long Trail, a 272-mile trail that runs through Vermont's Green Mountains from the Massachusetts state line to the Canadian border. We were supposed to be heading North on the Long Trail and instead we headed South. If I would have just stopped and looked at the signs at the trailhead or at my map, I would have known which way we were supposed to go. However, because I was stressed out about time, I didn't take the time to look. We lost over an hour and a half because I didn't stop to check the map, which would have taken less than a minute. We were able to hike Mount Abraham that day but we had to go back another day to hike Mount Ellen.

The bottom line is that, every once in a while, you want to slow down and check your map to make sure you're heading in the right direction. This is another reason writing down your goals is important. It'll serve as your map, to let you know whether you're still on track. By regularly coming back to check in on your progress, you can catch yourself quickly if you're heading in the wrong direction.

Activity

Get out your journal and write down the mantra: "A little progress each day adds up to big results." You may also want to write it on a notecard or a piece of paper where you can regularly see it. You *will* have days where you don't want to do the small daily disciplines that will get you closer to your goal. You *will* have days where you'll tell yourself that your effort isn't making any difference. This is why you need a tool in place to keep you on track when that nagging inner voice is trying to pull you back to the safety of your old comfort zone. This is where this mantra comes in.

Anytime you don't feel like doing your daily disciplines or you want to give up practicing a habit, repeat the mantra: "A little progress each day adds up to big results." Saying it over and over will help combat that inner voice that's pulling you in the wrong direction. It'll help nudge you into action or keep you going in the middle of an action so you can keep the ball rolling.

Another reason I love the book *The Compound Effect* by Darren Hardy is because it's based on the idea that simple disciplines, when practiced consistently, will compound overtime into significant results. He recognizes that most people give up on the simple disciplines when they don't see significant results right away. You must understand that, even though you may not see major results right away, sticking with the small disciplines will eventually yield results.

An interesting fact is, changing one aspect of your life can change other aspects of your life. For example, if you desire to get in shape, once you begin exercising consistently, you'll be more likely to start eating better. Likewise, once you begin changing your diet, you'll have more energy to exercise. Exercise often gives us more energy, particularly when practiced consistently. The additional energy will make you more alert at work and give you more energy to do other activities that will get you closer to other goals in your life. That's why you don't need to stress out about tackling multiple goals at once when you're just getting started. You'll see that the actions you take to improve one aspect of your life will naturally trickle into other aspects of your life.

Looming Deadlines

Having deadlines can help keep you on track, but don't get discouraged if it takes you longer to achieve your goal than you had originally anticipated. It's critical that you remain focused on your goal and not the obstacles that are hindering you from achieving your goal in your desired time frame. In *The Seven Spiritual Laws of Success*, Deepak Chopra discusses one-pointed intention. He states, "One-pointed intention means to hold your attention to the outcome that's intended with such unbending purpose that you absolutely refuse to put your attention on obstacles."[10] If you focus on the obstacles, you'll be more likely to get sidelined, go backward, or give up entirely.

Yes, facing obstacles on your journey will be difficult, and not hitting your initial deadline will be frustrating, but you can't let these frustrations fester for long. Just keep reminding yourself of why you began working toward this goal in the first place and what it would mean for you if you give up. I had to do this when I didn't finish my doctorate and my first book by the initial dates I set for myself. I ended up finishing both; I just needed to extend out the timeline for both goals because life threw unexpected obstacles in the way.

At first I was upset that I didn't reach my initial deadlines, but because I remained focused on my goals and not the obstacles that slowed me down, I was able to reach both of these goals. Although it's entirely possible that you'll complete your goal by your initial deadline, you must be mindful to not do so at the detriment of other aspects of your life. If your health and overall wellbeing are being jeopardized due to working toward your goal, I encourage you to slow down and consider pushing out your deadline.

When I was 37, I set the goal of being on Mount Everest on my 40th birthday. That was an enormous goal that required an immense amount of training and me to make a lot of money to pay for the expedition. Just the climb of Mount Everest would have cost me around $100,000, and that doesn't even include all the special gear I would need and all of the costs associated with traveling to different places to train for the climb. The process of reaching this goal not only began to break down my body, but it also began to break down my spirit. I began to dread going to the mountains because I knew I wouldn't be able to take time to enjoy the sights. I was going to carry a heavy pack and move at a fast pace to strengthen my body and mind. Unfortunately, it did the opposite. My joints and muscles began to ache more and more, and I began to lose my love for the mountains—the place where I first began to heal from my traumas.

When your deadlines begin hurting you, it's important to reevaluate why you chose that date in the first place. Most people set deadlines for their goals without having a good understanding of everything that would be involved in reaching that goal. I must admit that I randomly chose to be on Mount Everest when I turned

40 just because I liked the sound of it. It wasn't based on any form of reality.

Furthermore, not reaching my goal of completing my doctorate by the age of 23 sent me into a downward spiral of shame, depression, and suicidal thoughts. Since I already doubted myself and my abilities and I didn't meet the arbitrary deadline I set for myself, it just perpetrated that unending feeling that I was a failure. It took me a long time to learn that it's okay if I don't reach a goal in my desired time frame. I have since found the saying, "God's delays are not denials" to be very helpful when I feel that my goal is taking longer to achieve than expected or that I might not achieve it at all. Just because I don't achieve a goal right now doesn't mean that I never will. Maybe sometimes I'm meant to not achieve a certain goal so that I'll pivot and achieve an even bigger and better goal.

I wanted to inspire people by climbing the seven summits. I wanted to prove that all humans are capable of achieving difficult feats if only they set their mind to it. I wanted to show people that if I can achieve difficult goals, they can too. However, I realized that I don't need to keep climbing huge mountains to do this. I have multiple examples in my life of how I overcame tremendous adversity that I can share without spending tons of time and money and risking my life in the process.

My initial plan was to inspire people, not only from following my mountain climbing journey on social media, but also by writing books afterward that would inspire them. However, I realized that I can start writing about my life's journey on social media and in books right now, and that's what I've done. Instead of climbing Mount Everest by my 40th birthday, I published my first book when I was 39, and my second book (this book) will be published when I'm 40. I climbed a different type of mountain, and it still has inspired others. It didn't cost nearly as much money, take nearly as much time, and I didn't have to injure my body or risk my life in the process.

Similarly, I was crushed when I left chiropractic college because I never envisioned anything else for my life, but once I began to create a new identity for myself, a future with different possibilities, I was able to move forward. I've been blessed beyond measure since that time. Each pivot I've made since chiropractic college has enriched my life in a myriad of ways. I'm now grateful that I left chiropractic college. I feel that I'm on the exact path that I'm meant to be on. The same will hold true for you each time you're forced to pivot or push out a deadline for your goal.

Don't condemn yourself for where you are in your journey or for not moving faster, because every moment in your life is an opportunity to learn and grow. Every bit of wisdom and growth you'll experience along the way will prepare you for the next stage of your journey. Sometimes the growth you'll experience will cause you to transform into a different version of yourself, which will require a different set of goals to match the new you. Approach this new path with curiosity and excitement, and you'll find that you're no longer on a previous path for a reason. You outgrew it, and now you have new opportunities in front of you.

As you grow and change, you'll likely find that your previous goals no longer match the person you're becoming. You'll find that you can now consider goals that you previously never considered or didn't think were possible for you. The life I live now is not the one I initially envisioned for myself. It's better! That only happened because I was willing to adjust my previous deadlines and pivot when necessary. I encourage you to keep this in mind when you face obstacles in your journey. They may be exactly what you need to experience the growth you'll need to reach your intended goal, or to put you on a path to reach a goal that's even better for you.

Routines and Accountability

You must have a plan before pursuing your goal. After Stan died, my life was spiraling so out of control that I needed structure and routines. Many people are surprised about the significant focus I place on goal setting in the trauma healing journey, but it's because of how important it's been to me. After experiencing multiple traumas from a young age, I felt that I had very little control over anything in my life, but when I started to set goals for myself and get into regular routines, I began to feel as though I was taking back control of my days and ultimately my life.

I'm all about efficiency. Life is hard enough as it is, so I like to create systems that automate certain tasks so I can minimize how many decisions I must make each day. Routines decrease decision fatigue. They put specific practices on autopilot so that we can reserve our energy and focus on other tasks. I put everything on my calendar. Remember the Google Doc I mentioned in the beginning of this chapter that I titled "Daily Goals", I use it for everything from birthday reminders to reminders of when to change my sheets and towels. I put everything down to minimize how many things I must remember, think about, and make decisions about. I do it for both work and my personal life.

I use a Google Doc so I can access it anywhere from my phone or computer. I can cut and paste projects to move them to new dates. I copy and paste to repeat activities that occur over and over. I use strikethrough to indicate when I completed a project. It works really well for me. I find it more efficient than a paper calendar where you would need to physically write the same things over and over. But that's just me. I encourage you to find your own system that works for you.

I encourage you to put any steps you're going to take to reach your goal into your calendar so you're making sure to prioritize yourself each day. This is where the Google Sheet I mentioned in the beginning of this chapter that I titled "Daily Activities" comes in for me. I use it to mark off each day when I've completed certain tasks that are getting me closer to my goals. It feels so good to mark things off in my Google Sheet. It works well as an accountability system for me because I don't like having to mark that I didn't complete a task. For example, I use my Google Sheet to keep track of my goal of drinking two liters of fluid daily. I use a one liter Nalgene bottle that has measurements on the side so I can easily see where I'm at for the day. If I see it's early evening and I haven't reached a certain target on my bottle, I start downing the water so I don't have to mark "No" on the sheet to indicate that I didn't reach my daily goal.

Telling other people about your goals can help create a higher level of accountability. However, be careful who you share your goals with. If they feel that your goal isn't possible, they might try to discourage you. Oftentimes, this isn't meant to hurt you but to protect you from getting hurt. Also keep in mind that people aren't likely to encourage you to pursue something higher than what they've achieved or desire to achieve themselves. When a person's worldview is limited, and they don't expand it by learning about people that have achieved goals much greater than they have themselves, it'll be difficult for them to envision a different experience for you.

You must also be careful to not let yourself or anyone else paint you into a box. People get scared about saying their goals out loud because other people will likely check on their progress. This can be both good and bad. Being accountable to other people may keep you motivated on days you're feeling down, but it can also keep you in a box and make you feel as though you must continue pursuing that goal even if you know it's no longer the right path for you. I did this to myself when I put my goal out to the world that I was going to climb the seven summits and be on Mount Everest on my 40th birthday. Even when I felt that I no longer wanted to pursue this goal, I still kept moving forward to save face. I eventually decided to admit to the world that I was no longer interested in pursuing the goal. I could see the sheer disappointment in their faces when I told them that I was taking a break from the big mountains and rethinking my goals.

As I said in Chapter 4, many people like to live vicariously through me, so when I stopped my mountain adventures, I was also stopping their mountain adventures too. It's similar to when parents encourage their children to follow a career path that they had wanted for themselves. And when their child decides to not pursue that path, or starts the path and then abandons it for an alternate route, the parent often feels a deep sense of disappointment because they've lost the ability to watch their child achieve the goal they've coveted for so long.

These are all important things to keep in mind when you choose a goal and when you're deciding who you want to be involved in your journey toward achieving that goal. You must keep in mind that some people will be helpful to bring along the journey and others won't be. Some will keep you stuck on a path you don't want to be on and some will pull you off track so you don't climb higher than they're willing to go themselves. However, some will be cheering you on from the sidelines and will be there to give you encouragement when you're struggling to keep going. These are the people you want to bring along with you on your journey.

As a life coach, part of my job is to help keep my clients accountable on their path to achieving their goals, but the coaching relationship isn't meant to be a permanent one. I arm my clients with the tools they need to reach their goals and to be able to hold themselves accountable for the day when the coaching relationship ends. In the next activity, you'll learn to create your own plan for keeping yourself accountable.

Activity: Create an Accountability Plan

Get out your journal. Even if you won't use it to keep track of your progress, you'll use it to write down your accountability plan. First, write down where you'll record your goal and your desired time frame for reaching that goal so you can keep track of your progress. Will you use a notebook or a document on your phone or computer?

Even though you're starting with one goal, know that you'll add more goals later when you achieve the first one, or as you create sustainable habits toward your first goal. I've found using a living document helpful because it allows me to see my past goals, which reminds me of my ability to achieve the goals I set for myself. It also allows me to make edits to the document as my goals change or I change.

In your journal, write down how often you'll review your goals document to remind you of your goal and to make sure you're on track. For short-term goals (goals that will take less than six months to complete), I recommend you review the document once per week. For long-term goals (goals that will take more than six months to complete), I recommend you review the document once per month.

Next, write down in your journal people that you could ask to be your accountability partner or part of your accountability team. Choose people who will support you, encourage you to keep going when you feel defeated, and nudge you back on track when you've veered off course. Consider people that have similar goals as yours so you can support one another along the way.

As you start working toward more goals, you might find that you have different accountability partners for different goals. One friend and I had the same goal of decluttering our homes, and since we shared the same goal, we would regularly check in with each other to keep each other accountable for the goals we set for ourselves. We would also schedule regular video chats so we could be working on decluttering our homes at the same time and talk each other through a challenging part of the process. When my hiking partner and friend, Sarah and I are working toward a big hiking goal, we'll check in with each other in between hikes to make sure that we're staying consistent with the training we must do in between hikes.

If you would like to have the additional accountability from a coach, then start researching coaches. You could hire a life coach if you have multiple areas of your life that you want to work on. If you have fitness goals, you could hire a fitness coach. If you have relationship goals, you could hire a relationship coach. You can go onto Google and search for coaches in your area or online coaches.

Another way to hold yourself accountable is by announcing your goal to your social media followers and then commit to regularly post about your progress on your social media page. You could also post when you're having a bad day or when you slip up on your progress. You may find the support and encouragement from your friends and followers helpful in keeping you on track or getting you back on track.

It's important to have a plan in place on how you're going to achieve your goal and ways to hold yourself accountable, but you must remain flexible and open to alternate routes to achieving your goal. I'm prone to being rigid, so I must regularly remind myself to not be resistant to new ideas and alternate paths to success. I was taken aback when I read what James Redfield wrote about Type A people who are obsessed with their work and can't slow down, in his book, *The Celestine Prophecy*. He said, "They can't slow down because they use their routine to distract themselves, to reduce life to only its practical considerations. And they do this to avoid recalling how uncertain they are about why they live."[11] This hit close to home for me.

Part of why I love pursuing goals is because it provides me with a distraction to avoid thoughts from my past or uncertainties about my future, which often creep in when I slow down. I also want so much for my existence to matter. After years of being made to feel that I was unimportant and insignificant, I'm now on this quest to prove otherwise to my victimizers and ultimately to myself. However, this has come with a great cost because I still haven't embraced the idea for myself that being good enough is enough.

Each new goal I reach only gives me a moment's relief from the feeling that I'm not enough. Very quickly, my nagging inner critic tells me that it's still not enough and I must accomplish more. I can't condemn this part of me because it's served me; I've accomplished a lot in my life, but I must regularly keep this part of me in check. I don't want to stop working hard to achieve new goals because the process is exciting to me, and many of my goals are focused on serving others. It's just that I must always stay on guard of pushing toward a goal to the point where I let other aspects of my life start to fall apart. So, that's also part of my own personal accountability system. I not only make sure that I'm on track to reaching my goal but I also make sure that I'm not criticizing myself for not being farther along.

I take the time to celebrate my wins and to celebrate myself. That inner wound of feeling that I'm not enough runs deep—so deep that I'm not sure if it'll ever fully heal. So, I must always take time to clean that wound of debris that could cause it to open back up or slow down its healing. That debris is made up of my negative self-talk and memories from my past that have crept back in.

If you share these same types of wounds and same type of debris that keep your wounds open and raw, I encourage you to hold yourself accountable and celebrate your small wins along the way. Small wins can be taking a step toward reaching your goal that was hard but you did it anyway. It can be a milestone that signifies that you're getting closer to your goal. I encourage you to celebrate even the fact that you haven't given up on your goal and yourself, because that is surely a win!

Chapter 6
Continuous Improvement

You must constantly look for opportunities to improve. This is because in every aspect of life, we're either growing or dying. We may reach what appears to be a plateau, but it's just an illusion and it's easy to slide back and lose ground. I've experienced this myself with my lifelong battle with my weight. It can take me only weeks to put on 20 pounds, but it'll take me months or years to get it off. That's why you must continuously take steps to reach your goal, whether it's actual physical steps, or changing your mindset and constantly motivating yourself to do the work necessary to reach your goal.

When we get too comfortable in our current circumstances, we're likely to get blindsided when our relationships, career, and health start to decline out of nowhere. We feel the decline happened suddenly when in reality it started the moment we took our foot off the gas and thought we were just coasting. Even if you have a great relationship with your partner, you can always make it better. Even if you're good at your job and enjoy it, you can always improve yourself and enjoy it even more. Even if you're physically in great shape, there's always room for improvements.

Think of money. If you save your money for retirement in a typical, low interest savings account, its value will gradually decline due to inflation. That's why you must invest the money so it can grow over time. The same thing happens with our health. As we get older, the breakdown of our cells occurs at a faster rate than the replacement and repair of those cells. Therefore, if we're not constantly working on improving our diet and our level of activity, our health gradually declines.

Take your muscles for example. If you stop working them, they'll gradually diminish in size, lose their strength, and lose their ability to contract and sustain activity for extended periods of time. The same thing happens with your brain. If you're not constantly stimulating your brain, you'll begin to lose neural connections in your brain, and its function will decline. Our body is focused on conserving resources. So if you're not constantly utilizing parts of your brain or other parts of your body, then your body isn't going to maintain that tissue. Now you see why it's important that you keep improving yourself.

Continuous improvement may sound overwhelming, but in practice, it only needs to be small, incremental improvements. Once you create habits surrounding different aspects of your life, you just need to keep doing them and push yourself a little further over time. Once your activities become habits, it's not difficult to improve them. For example, if you're already exercising and dedicating a certain amount of time to it, it becomes easy to increase the weight you're lifting or increase your speed when walking or running. You can improve without putting in extra time.

People often get overwhelmed at just the thought of continuous improvement because they think it means a greater time investment. However, if you're already investing time into your relationships, career, and health every day, then it's not going to be difficult to include incremental improvements over time. Just take what you've been doing and tweak it a little bit so you're pushing yourself a little bit more and becoming a little bit better with each progressing month and year of your life.

You must continue to do the work you did to achieve the goal in the first place, even after the goal has been achieved. If you stop taking steps, you're going to slide back. This is why all diets work, but all diets also fail. If people follow the protocols for any diet, they'll lose weight. However, once the weight is shed and they stop the diet, all the weight comes back and sometimes even more. If the diet is highly restrictive, it most likely won't be sustainable. People usually won't keep up the diet after they've reached their weight loss goal, then they resume their previous eating patterns and they put all the weight back on.

I love Tony Robbins' saying: "Do what you did in the beginning of a relationship and there won't be an end." This concept applies to all aspects of our life. It's very common that we stop doing what strengthened our relationship in the first place. We stop being the best employee. Instead of being grateful for our job, we start to think we're owed more than we're being given and slack off because of it. We want the body we had when we were young and active but we don't want to do the work to get back in shape and maintain it.

If you used to enjoy your work, what can you do to feel that way again, even if you're planning on pursuing another job in the future? If you think you want a new relationship, what can you do to rekindle old flames before you call it quits? If you do the same thing in the next relationship (start off strong and fizzle out), that relationship will also come to an end. If you were once at a level of physical fitness you desired, how can you get back to that level or even better?

We make excuses of what someone else is or isn't doing. We make excuses for our metabolisms being slower or not having as much time. We make excuses for our finances not being better because we're not making enough money or taxes being too high, but we forget that by blaming everyone and everything else for our undesirable circumstances, we're giving our power away. We're not taking responsibility and control over our life. It doesn't matter how bad your life has been to this point, you always have the ability to change your future circumstances. Sometimes it requires a mindset shift. Sometimes it requires setting goals and taking action to achieve them, and many times it requires both a mindset shift and getting clear about your goals. There's no exception when it comes to healing from trauma. You'll continuously need to improve the way you think.

I know people who spend decades of their life being resentful and angry about their trauma, not understanding why it happened to them, and focusing on all that they've lost and will no longer be. They literally give decades of their life away to something that can't be changed. Yes, our traumas caused us pain. Yes, it sucks that we had to endure everything. Yes, there are people who were wrong for hurting us and not doing more to protect us, but there's not a single thing that can be done to change any of that. And that's exactly my point!

I'm not saying that a person is wrong for feeling pain and resentment, because I understand why those feelings arise and I've experienced those feelings myself. What I am saying is that there's not a thing we can do about our past circumstances. The longer we focus on our past that can't be changed, the longer we'll be stuck. This is why I emphasize the importance of reading and listening to personal and professional development resources. It's been absolutely critical in getting me unstuck and helping me persevere through the difficult times in my life. I want you to know that it can be just as effective in your life.

I've always been into personal development, but I started making it a daily practice in the beginning of 2018, and my life has never been better. Each year continues to be better than the last. It doesn't mean that I don't have hard days and I don't have to do any more work to heal and improve the way I experience life. Life is always going to be hard, and there's always going to be more work that needs to be done. However, the way I'm experiencing life and my relationships and the satisfaction I get out of life is compounding every single year because of the way I'm changing, the way I'm growing, and the way my view of the world has evolved. I'm now looking at things with a different lens. And by continuously improving myself, I'm continuously changing how I look at myself, others, and my circumstances, which means I experience life in a completely different way. I can open up the possibilities of how I look at my trauma and other circumstances that were out of my control.

As I said in Chapter 4, I love to use reframing to change how I look at a situation, behavior, habit, or circumstance. I saw that I could either continue to focus on what I didn't have control over and stay stuck in feelings of hopelessness and helplessness, or I could focus on what was in my control. What I did have control over, what I could change, is the way I thought about myself and past circumstances. These shifts in thinking moved me into a position of power. I felt in control over my thoughts instead of having my thoughts control me. By reading and listening to the stories of people who've done tremendous things after their trauma, I realized that it's possible to lead a highly productive life and serve the world in enormous ways after one's trauma. It's empowering and exciting to know that someone out there has thrived after their trauma, and if they could do it, then you and I can do it too!

I still spend one to three hours daily on personal or professional development. Some of the time is spent reading books or articles. Some of it is spent completing activities for a new professional certification I'm working on. Most of it's spent listening to audiobooks so I can be learning while I'm doing other activities. I listen to audiobooks when I'm getting dressed for the day, cleaning, driving, or getting ready for bed at night. Not only does it provide me with different insights and perspectives but it also helps me stay focused on my goal. If I'm working on a financial goal, I'll listen to books on finance. If I'm working on a business goal, I'll listen to books about business success. As the Book of Ecclesiastes in the Bible says, "There is no new thing under the sun." This means that others have gone before you and have charted the path you're looking to embark on yourself.

It's very common for people to stay surrounded by people who think like them and to only look at information that supports their current point of view, but if you're only surrounding yourself with people and information that aligns with your current way of thinking, you're never going to change. There won't be anything to force you outside of your comfort zone and what you currently know to be true about life. This is why I love meeting new people. I love traveling to different countries and talking with people that live in a different culture than I do. Being a consummate learner has opened up new ways of thinking that weren't possible to me when I was only looking inward and cycling through the existing thoughts that were in my head. With new input, I could see life from a different perspective. This excited me, filled me with hope, and made me feel that I wasn't going to be trapped in the pain of my trauma forever.

I'm not always taking in new information. I often revisit concepts I'm familiar with in books I've already listened to. Even if I've listened to the same book many times, I always glean something new from it each time I relisten. As time goes on, I'm different, and so is my frame of mind. This means that I'll be more open to ideas that I might not have been ready to receive in the past. Relistening to books that previously resonated with me can also reinforce that I'm on the right path, nudge me back on track when I've gotten off course, or remind me that there's more work to be done and that the work number stops.

As I said in Chapter 2, mentors are invaluable. Some of my mentors are people I know personally, who've achieved success in areas of life where I want to achieve success. Some of my mentors are no longer alive, but I can access their teachings through books and other resources they left behind. I can also access mentors who are alive but I may never meet, through their books and resources. Whenever I can, I go to conferences and join online workshops to see my mentor in person or virtually.

The next activity will provide you with the opportunity to brainstorm people who could be your mentor, regardless of whether you'll ever have the opportunity to meet them. I encourage you to expand your current reality by researching people who've achieved your desired goals. Many people don't pursue certain goals because they think it's impossible for them and it's not part of their current reality. So, if you want to start a business, for example, and you have very little money to invest, then it's important to read books, listen to podcasts, or watch YouTube videos on starting a business with little money. By taking the time to research the topic surrounding your goal, you'll be able to find people that were once in your predicament. You'll realize that, if they could achieve it, then you can achieve it too.

Activity

Research mentors for your goal. Make a list of people in your life that have achieved success in the area of your life you're looking to improve. Tell them about your goal, how their success has inspired you, and ask them if they would be willing to talk with you about how they did it. Be willing to be flexible. This individual may not have a lot of time available. So, let them know that you respect their time and you won't take up too much of their time. They might be willing to talk on the phone or meet for lunch. Whatever is most convenient for them.

I've found that the more successful a person is, the more willing they are to mentor others. It's because mentors have been so important in their journey that they now want to pay it forward. My mentors have been very gracious with their time, but you don't want to make the assumption that they will be right out of the gate. Most mentors want to evaluate your level of commitment to your goal and to yourself before they put a lot of their own time into you. Don't expect someone to dedicate more time to help you reach your goal than you're willing to put into it yourself.

I encourage you to make use of the wealth of free resources that are out there on the Internet to help research your goal. If you don't know where to begin, Google is a great place to start. Research what it would take to start your own business, the college degree you want to pursue, the athletic competition you want to engage in, or whatever your goal may be. Research people who've achieved your desired goal, and gather the books and other resources that detail how they did it. Use your research to develop your plan of action.

Start making playlists on YouTube and finding books and podcasts that are related to the topic of your goal. This way you can have resources ready anytime you need a shot of motivation to keep moving forward. For my YouTube videos, I put them in a playlist I named "P & P Development" meaning "Personal and Professional Development", but you can give your playlist any name of your choice. As you're reading or listening to new information, pay attention to when they discuss people and books that have influenced them. Look them up immediately or make a note to look them up later. I always want to know who influenced the people I admire. I then go and learn from those same people, knowing that they'll likely impact me in a similar way.

I was recently at the bank to open a business checking account. When I told the branch manager that I was opening accounts at different banks because I'll be using the Profit First method that I've been learning about, she looked at me surprised and said,

"You're a life coach and you're still learning?" I looked at her stunned and replied, "Always. I never stop learning." I spent 12 years in college, I taught over 20 different courses during my 12 years as a college professor, and I still dedicate one to three hours to personal and professional development every day. I never stop learning, and I never will. I encourage you to think of learning in the same way.

Learning accelerates our ability to change. It stretches our view of what's possible. It allows us to think about ways we can escape the box that's kept us trapped in a life that we don't enjoy. However, we must do more than just listen to audio and read books and articles. As John Maxwell says in *Developing the Leader Within You 2.0*, "Application stimulates transformation. Nothing happens with information unless it's applied."[12] We must take action on what we're learning. That's why throughout this book I've provided you with activities so you're not only learning, but you can apply the concepts to your life immediately.

Tame Your Inner Critic

I was walking into the classroom to teach anatomy and physiology when I heard a student talking about her "big" ass. I stopped and said, "I don't allow negative self-talk in my classroom." She quickly retorted, "But it's true. I'm just stating something that's true about myself." I replied, "Do you tell yourself all the other things that are true about yourself—that you're smart, you're beautiful, you're a great mom, and you're a great wife? Do you tell yourself those *truths* as well, or do you only tell yourself your negative *truths*?"

We are our own worst critics. We judge ourselves harshly and then wonder why we don't feel confident of achieving our desired goals. How are you going to achieve great things if you keep telling yourself that you're ugly, stupid, or you don't understand math, science, or any new topic you're trying to learn? How are you going to ever achieve your goals if you keep focusing on your shortcomings? You must start focusing on your gifts, what's good about you, and what you have to offer the world. And don't tell me you don't have any gifts or special skills because we all do. We just don't give ourselves enough credit for the areas in life where we shine.

You must constantly improve on your self-talk so you can keep your inner critic at bay. You must become aware of the things you regularly say to yourself that keep you down. I'm not saying not to recognize your faults, we all have them. What I am saying is that you must also focus on the good about you because you're never going to feel empowered or strong enough to overcome your faults if you don't feel you have enough strengths to compensate for your weaknesses. You may not feel good enough to achieve the goals you want to achieve. You may not think you're pretty enough to get the relationship you're looking for. You may not think you're smart enough to go after the job or business that you want to pursue. Focusing on your negatives is only going to keep you small. It's easy to blame external forces for our inadequacies, but the reality is that we keep ourselves small by the way we talk to ourselves and by our limiting beliefs.

Our core beliefs are our most deeply held beliefs about ourselves and the world. We acquired them as children, before the age of seven. Therefore, it's very difficult to get rid of them because they've become part of our identity. As we progress through life, we acquire more limiting beliefs that reinforce our deeply held core beliefs. When we were children, we couldn't decipher what was true and what wasn't. We took in everything that was said to us as truth because we depended on the people around us to explain to us how the world works and how we fit into the world.

As children, we took what our parents, teachers, religious leaders, and community leaders said as gospel because they were grown and we thought they must know best. We go through the rest of our lives with these beliefs that were ingrained in us by people that never worked on expanding their horizons. If only we knew that they were also limited by their own beliefs. If only we could see that our parents were dealing with unresolved pains from their own childhoods. If only we knew that our teachers said things based on their own limiting beliefs and were under an immense amount of stress because they were overworked and underpaid. If only we knew!

As we grew older, we held onto these limiting beliefs, and then we started to collect evidence of why they're true, which further ingrained them in our mind. It's just like an internet search; most people don't look at conflicting opinions and try to think about which one makes more sense, they only look at the information that supports their belief before the internet search. This is how the Internet reinforces false beliefs in the minds of people. Although the Internet has an abundant amount of information, some of it can be inaccurate. The same goes for social media. So it's really important that we learn to think critically. We must learn to question not only information that comes into us from the outside world but also the internal beliefs that are holding us back.

Although most of our core beliefs were implanted in our mind during childhood by the people around us, it's now our responsibility as adults to undo the damage that was done to us by them. This is where I encourage you to use reframing. These people have given us an obstacle to overcome, but our greatest potential for growth comes from the most difficult experiences in our life. Think about the type of person you'll become once you're able to overcome the baggage you've been lugging around for most of your life. Imagine the sense of relief you'll feel when you finally set the baggage down and walk away. Your hands, feet, and body are already stressed from carrying the baggage for so long, and the farther away you get from the baggage, the more those injuries will heal, and the better you'll feel.

Even though we have all these things working against us, it's our responsibility to override these negative beliefs. This is where many people go wrong. Because it's usually other people that planted the seeds of self-doubt and self-criticism in our minds, we think it's their job to rid us of the negativities by telling us how much they love us, how much they appreciate us, how great we are, and how much our existence matters. However, it's our job to make ourselves feel better about ourselves. I'm not saying we shouldn't look to be in relationships with people that elevate us and make us feel better about ourselves. I'm saying that we shouldn't depend on another person to pull up the weeds that have taken over our emotional garden. It's our garden, and it's up to us to pull up each weed and keep doing it each time it grows back.

You must also begin to question the source of your beliefs and not holding onto every thought in your mind as pure gospel. Just because it's in your mind doesn't mean it's true. That's why an upcoming activity will allow you to begin challenging your negative beliefs. When you begin to look for evidence to the contrary, it begins to open your mind to new possibilities. It'll allow you to envision a future that's different from your past or current reality.

Before we move into the next activity, it's important to understand that all the people that have hurt us, whether intentionally or unintentionally, did so because of the pain they've experienced in their own lives. It doesn't mean that what they did was okay, it means that the beliefs we acquired from them are likely not true. All the times people told us that we weren't good enough, smart enough, or pretty enough were likely a reflection of the pain they experienced in the past and the way they were currently feeling about themselves. Instead of inwardly reflecting upon their pain, they were outwardly expressing their pain onto us. You must know this so you can begin to let go of the beliefs you've acquired from the people around you and your trauma. Once you understand this, it'll be easier to find examples in your life of where the negative beliefs you have about yourself are false.

Yes, sometimes you procrastinate, get angry, don't look your best, or can't focus, but that doesn't mean that these things are always true. As a professor, it was so hard for me to hear students say, "I'm not a good student", "I'm not a good test-taker", "I'm not good at science." I knew these limiting beliefs they had about themselves were holding them back in class. When I had the opportunity to question them further on their beliefs, I would ask them to look for evidence to the contrary. For example, if they said, "I'm not a good test-taker," I would ask them to identify points in their life where they have passed an exam. Then I would point out that they wouldn't be in college if they hadn't passed a lot of exams. They were usually surprised at this argument. The reality is that we say we're not good at something based on what we were told many years ago, and because we believe it to be true, we ignore all the evidence to the contrary, much like we do in an internet search. That's why I encourage you to start collecting evidence to the contrary and begin challenging your long-held beliefs that are keeping you playing small in your life.

Another thing I learned about human nature by listening to and watching my students is, people naturally gravitate toward their strengths and avoid their weaknesses. My students would put most of their energy into assignments and classes that they liked and knew they could do really well in. Then they would put off working on the classes that they didn't like or feel successful in because they had negative beliefs about their learning ability. Most of them were going into nursing or other healthcare programs. I was teaching them foundational courses like anatomy and physiology. They put so much energy into other courses like English, psychology and sociology that they didn't have a lot of extra time for my class. They would spend their time studying for my class on a lab quiz that was worth five percent of their grade instead of focusing on studying for a lecture exam that was worth fifteen percent of their grade. They didn't want to feel like a failure, so they focused on the classes and assignments that they knew they could do well in. The issue is that they ultimately ended up further anchoring their beliefs that they're not a good test taker or they're not good at science. They would score poorly on the lecture exams, not because they weren't capable but because they focused their energies elsewhere. They avoided their weaknesses, and by doing so, they further solidified in their mind that there was no point in trying. It became a self-fulfilling prophecy.

Where have you done this in your own life? My coaching clients regularly do it with their weight loss efforts. Research has found time and time again that exercise has little impact on weight loss in comparison to changing your diet. Yet many people who begin a weight loss journey (including myself) gravitate toward physical activity for weight loss instead of focusing on their diet. Changing your diet is hard, so many people gravitate toward what they think will be the easier way to lose weight, which is through exercise. However, it becomes just another self-fulfilling prophecy.

People don't realize that one of two things happen when they start burning extra calories through exercise: they either begin to eat more to compensate for the calories lost through exercise, or they don't eat more and their body lowers its basal metabolic rate (BMR). This means that your body will require fewer calories during exercise and during your daily activities. Ultimately, both options lead to little weight loss and eventually a weight plateau. It ingrains in your mind that you can't lose weight, so you stop exercising. And since you've further ingrained in your mind that you can't lose weight, you don't do the hard work, but the essential work, of tackling your diet. You figure, what's the point?

Author, Kelly Lee Phipps, is commonly quoted as saying, "If you argue for your limitations, you get to keep them. But if you argue for your possibilities, you get to create them!" It's so easy for people who've experienced trauma to fall into this same trap that my students and clients fell into. They ruminate over what they've lost and what will never be possible. I fell into this trap myself, but

I'm also proof that there's always a way out of this trap. Instead of fighting to prove your limitations to be true, fight to prove that your biggest goals are possible. Our brains have amazing capabilities. We can master whatever we put our mind to. Our brain will grow stronger connections the more we practice a new skill. This is why it's important to tame your inner critic. It's a difficult task but not an impossible one.

On August 19, 2021, I participated in the workshop, Trauma & the Journey to Wholeness: Art Making and Healing, led by Sheryl Kaplan and Judith Prest at the Wiawaka Center for Women in Lake George, New York. One of the activities for the day was to depict our inner critic. We were provided with an abundant amount of clippings from magazines to choose from to create a collage that would best represent our inner critic. I knew that I had to find the most vicious pictures possible for my inner critic. I chose a wolf growling with its teeth showing, a walrus with a bloody face, and two wolves ripping apart an animal. They appropriately represented how brutal my inner critic is. I knew I needed teeth and blood showing in my inner critic because I feel like I'm being ripped apart when my inner critic is at work. It's breaking me down and destroying me piece by piece.

One thing that many people are surprised to hear about me is that I'm very insecure about my level of intelligence. There is a part of me that doesn't believe that I'm smart because, as a child, I was told that I wasn't smart and that I would never amount to anything. As I said in Chapter 1, I had chronic ear infections as a child that damaged my hearing. It took time for my family, teachers, and doctors to realize that I wasn't doing well in school because I couldn't hear my teachers. Once they figured it out, they had me start sitting in the front of the class so I could hear them. I did extra work to correct problems with my speech and concentrate in my classes. However, I'll never forget the many times I was called dumb and stupid. Even though I was Salutation of my senior class in high school, I completed my PhD, and I taught over 20 different courses on the college level, there's still a part of me that thinks that I'm dumb and stupid. It's part of my inner critic that's continually gnawing on me and I'm continually having to do the work of bandaging up the gaping wounds it's created.

I brainstormed a ferocious name for my inner critic with the group I was in, and we came up with "Diablo", which is the Spanish word for devil. The moment someone said it, I knew it was the perfect representation of my inner critic. I wrote the name "Diablo" on a piece of paper so I could paste it along with the pictures on my collage. Since that time, I'm convinced of the importance of putting a name to one's inner critic, and I recommend you do the same so you can call it out by its name when it's at work.

The last image I included on my collage was of a large, adult gorilla that was looking down from a tree. The face on the gorilla made me feel like it was looking down with judgment and condemnation. This is also part of my inner critic. I can be very judgmental and hard on myself, and that's a reflection of the voice from my inner critic condemning my every move and judging everything I say. Even though I've done a lot of great work and my inner critic isn't as loud as it used to be, it still comes rearing its ugly head every now and then. Again, this inner critic developed early, and the more traumas I experienced, the more ferocious it became.

To combat this vicious inner critic, I began to puff up my ego to try prove my inner critic wrong. In an effort to not be judged so harshly by it, I tried to become great at as many things as I could. I inflated my ego by pursuing big degrees, big titles, and big adventures that people would be impressed by. However, this drove me into perfectionism, which set me up for more failure because nothing I could do would fully measure up to the expectations of my inner critic. My inner critic could always point out some fault, something that I did wrong, something I could have done better, or how I'm not as good as someone else.

Creating a visual representation of my inner critic was so beneficial to me, and I recommend you do the same. By visually seeing how brutal my inner critic is, it allowed me to be more compassionate to myself whenever it's at work. I realized why it's so difficult to tame, why it always comes out to play when I'm already feeling weak, and why it's easier for my inner critic to win and harder for me to stay in the battle when life is beating me down. You could create a collage like I did, or you could paint it or draw it. You could also search on the Internet for pictures and create a digital one on your phone or computer.

Additionally, I encourage you to give a name to your inner critic and talk out loud to it. The voice of your inner critic can get so loud that sometimes the only way to overpower it is to talk out loud to it. However, I don't recommend you do this when in the presence of others. Society doesn't look favorably on people who talk to themselves, and especially on people who talk to voices inside their head. But if your inner critic is anything like mine, it's most active when you're by yourself, and it comes out to play when you're still. If it begins to rear its ugly head when you're by yourself, that's the perfect time to tell it to quiet down. Once you do this, I encourage you to spend additional time talking directly to the wounded part of yourself that feels that it must cower in the presence of your inner critic. For example, I say things like, "You're okay, Steph. You're okay. You're safe right now." It's like I'm comforting my inner child that doesn't feel safe in that moment and didn't feel safe all those times in my life that I was being hurt and programmed by others.

It's easy to be hard on ourselves for our negative self-talk, but it's important to remember that we've had a lot more actual voices in our life telling us all the ways that we're no good and that our existence doesn't matter than we've had positive voices telling us that we are good and that we do matter. That's why trauma can be so devastating; it can reinforce negative beliefs that we already have about ourselves, or it can push us to use negative coping strategies that put us in situations that can hurt us.

There will always be scars left behind from the damage that was done by our parents, teachers, society, and victimizers. That's why it'll take constant work to keep your nagging inner critic at bay. One thing that's helped me is to think about the quote by Greek poet, Dinos Christianopoulos who said, "They tried to bury us, but they didn't know we were seeds." So many times, people have tried to bury me. They've tried to make me feel small and as though my existence didn't matter, but what they didn't realize is that I was a seed. The pain and humiliation they exacted upon me didn't destroy me. Instead, they provided me with the fertile ground I needed to grow and thrive. Again, this is why I titled my first book, *Transformation After Trauma*, because that's truly what's possible after experiencing trauma, a *transformation*. We're all seeds that can flourish after being buried.

As I said in Chapter 4, they're called limiting beliefs because they limit us. To experience a transformation, you'll need to tackle these long-held beliefs, as they'll be the most likely culprits in preventing your success. You won't aim for something more if you have a belief that you're not smart enough, pretty enough, or simply not enough. Think about what would be possible for you if you were to change your narrative. Who would you be and how would your life be different if you replace those beliefs with ones that are more useful to you? The purpose of the next activity is for you to challenge your limiting beliefs and finally break free from them.

Activity: Discovering the Real Truth

Go back to the list of limiting beliefs surrounding your chosen goal that you wrote down in the beginning of Chapter 4. On a new page in your journal, write down each limiting belief. You can add newly identified limiting beliefs in the journal as well.

Now look at each limiting belief one by one and write down examples of when they were *not* true. For example, if you have the limiting belief that you can't trust anyone, then write down examples of when people showed you they were trustworthy. Of course you're going to have examples of when people weren't trustworthy, but that's not the point of this activity. The point is for you to see that, even though something may be true in one aspect of your life or may have been true in the past, it doesn't mean that it is or will always be true. You're looking for evidence to point to when you start saying these limiting beliefs so you can stop sabotaging yourself.

If you're looking to strengthen your relationship with your significant other, or enter a new relationship, or you're looking to improve your relationships with your family and friends, how on Earth are you going to be able to do that if you believe that no one can be trusted? You'll always be guarded and only give a part of yourself in relationships. The point of this exercise is to make you more resourceful so you don't feel stuck moving forward. If your current beliefs aren't serving you and will hinder your progress, I'm providing you with a way to start challenging them so they don't keep holding you down.

Do you have a goal to improve your financial situation but have the belief that you're not good with money? If so, start looking for evidence of when you've made good decisions with money. Do you have a goal to lose weight but you have the belief that you can't lose weight? If so, start looking for evidence of when you've lost some weight in the past. Don't undo this by saying, "But I gained the weight back, so that doesn't count." No, it does count! It's your limiting beliefs that caused you to gain back the weight in the first place. You're looking for ammunition so you can fight against this part of you that wants to keep drawing you back into your not so comfortable, comfort zone.

You must keep in mind the widely attributed quote, "What gets rewarded gets repeated." If you reward your limiting beliefs by supplying them with more examples of their truth, they'll strengthen and continue to reverberate in your mind. However, if you instead look for evidence to the contrary, overtime it can override your limiting beliefs so your new beliefs become predominant. Therefore, as you move forward in the coming days and weeks, continue to look for evidence in your current life where your limiting beliefs were proven untrue in different situations, and make note of it in your journal.

Your inner critic can easily sabotage your success. Even when you set a goal and start making progress toward it, be prepared for when your inner critic will come rearing its ugly head. It'll likely be at the times when you're already feeling down and discouraged. It knows when you're most vulnerable and when it can have its greatest effect. You must prepare for those times by maintaining consistent personal growth and development and getting familiar with the words that will be most effective to combat the voice in your head when you're in that dark place.

Fill Your Mind With Positivity

Every once in a while when I'm walking, I like to put out my arms, close my eyes for a brief moment, and focus on the sun and breeze on my skin. It always makes me smile. Being surrounded by all elements of nature makes me feel alive and reminds me how blessed I am. When I'm home, I like to place my hands on my chest so I can feel my heartbeat. I'm so grateful that it's still beating. I'm so grateful that I hung on and didn't give up. This simple practice fills me with gratitude and joy.

Of course I still have difficult days from time to time, but I'm generally happy and cheery, and I like to look at the bright side of everything. I know that the people who only see this side of me probably think I'm a Pollyanna, but I'm not. I know that life is hard, and right around the corner could be just another tragedy waiting to happen. But what point is there in not enjoying the moments of joy as they come? Even if they're fleeting, why can't we embrace them? If we don't, all we'll be doing is focusing on all the bad that's happened and preparing for the next shoe to drop. That's a hard way to live if you ask me, but sadly that's the way many people have chosen to live. I'm asking you to choose a different way. I'm asking you to embrace beauty, joy, and happiness, regardless of how brief the encounters may be. I've had a tremendous amount of pain in my life, so I can always find reasons that life is hard, but I'm committed to not experiencing suffering every single day. I've made the choice to experience love, joy, and beauty because it's a much more enjoyable way to live. You can make the same choice.

Every day, you must look for ways to remind yourself that life is beautiful. The media and the news know that humans have a negativity bias, meaning that we're more likely to pay attention to negative news and negative information. It's an evolutionary instinct we have. We always want to be on the lookout for danger so we can survive. Unfortunately, our brain doesn't have the same pull toward positive information as it does for negative information.

News outlets don't focus on positive, uplifting stories, because they know our brains aren't as interested in them, and they won't maintain the ratings they need to stay in business. This affects our daily lives as we constantly live in fear of unknown danger and become paranoid that something bad might happen to us. Our minds overlook anything that's positive because it's totally focused on the negative. We're constantly bombarded with negativity in our lives so much that it takes constant conscious effort to make our mind aware of the good around us.

As the popular quote goes, "What you feed grows. What you starve dies." If you begin to feed your mind with positive thoughts, your negative thoughts will begin to fall away. Although they won't disappear forever. Think of them like a hearty weed, you can pull it out, but invariably there will always be a tiny root left behind. Once it's fed again, it begins to grow. Likewise, tiny roots of our negative beliefs will remain intact and we'll need to remain vigilant to starve them of the nutrients—the negative thoughts—they need to grow. When they do emerge above ground again, you need to pull them while they're little so they don't choke out the new growth of positive thoughts that you replaced them with.

As Tony Robbins often says, "Kill the monster while it's little." This means you want to build an arsenal to fight your negative thoughts. You should fill your mind with positive inputs from what you watch, read, and listen to. You want to think and say positive things about yourself. You also want to watch what you're saying about other people. Each time you talk negatively about a person, it anchors those beliefs about that person in your mind. So, it'll be more difficult over time to find the good in that person because you're only focusing on the bad. The same is true about the way you talk negatively about yourself.

During my years of teaching about the human body, I always got most excited when teaching about the brain. A part of the brain that's particularly fascinating is the reticular activating system (RAS). It acts as a filter; only the information that's important to us and our survival gets through. Our brain is bombarded every second of the day with stimuli from our internal and external environment. Our brain can't take time to process every bit of information coming in because it wouldn't be able to focus on the activities that are most important to our survival. So the RAS only allows in the information that we need to survive, as well as what we tell our brain is important.

A good example of the RAS in action is when you're going to buy something new like a car. Once you choose a new vehicle, you'll start seeing that same vehicle everywhere. It happened when I first bought my Honda CR-V. Before I bought it, I never noticed CR-Vs because I never told my brain that it was important, but the moment I started looking at buying a CR-V, I saw CR-Vs everywhere I went. This doesn't mean that everyone started buying CR-Vs at the same time as me. The other CR-Vs were always there, I just didn't notice them because my RAS filtered out that information because it deemed it unimportant.

This same concept applies to the thoughts we think about ourselves, other people, our trauma, our ability to move forward, and life in general. Therefore, if we tell our brain that we only want to focus on everything that's wrong with us, other people, and the world, that's what it'll do because we're telling our RAS to let that information through. However, if we tell our brain to focus on everything that's good about us, other people, and the world, it'll do that instead.

One idea for training your RAS to focus on positivity instead of negativity is to start your day with a gratitude practice and not with scrolling through social media, the news, text messages, or email. When you start your day with negative news and other people's priorities, you're letting the rest of the world dictate what your day is going to look like. Your gratitude practice doesn't need to be long. You can say out loud or write down three people or things you're grateful for and why, before you get out of bed. You can also do other things such as meditation, yoga, reading or listening to positive and uplifting resources like books and podcasts. The important thing is that you take control of your days by taking control of your mornings.

The same goes with how you end your day. I don't encourage you to end your day with looking at anything that can hijack your thoughts before you go to bed, such as social media, the news, email, or violent movies or TV shows. Instead, you could meditate. There are many apps like Insight Timer with guided meditations including ones that will prepare you for sleep. You could read or listen to a positive or uplifting book, or you could say or write down three to five wins or positive experiences you had during your day. Whatever it is, it should be something positive. You must remember that these are going to be the last thoughts on your mind before you go to bed.

The information you take in before going to bed could affect how quickly you fall asleep, how long you stay asleep, and the quality of your sleep. Getting good sleep is very important because poor sleep quality can have a negative impact on your day and your overall quality of life. It affects the way your body feels, your mood, and your ability to focus. It'll be difficult to start your day with positivity if you feel like crap. That's why it's important to alter the inputs in your mind right before you go to bed and right after you wake up in the morning. I'm not saying you should never go on social media, look at the news, or watch TV or movies with violence. I'm encouraging you to minimize your inputs from those sources and protect yourself from them when you first wake up and right before you go to bed.

I want you to know that you'll never be able to fully prevent yourself from having negative experiences and thoughts, and you'll have sleepless nights from time-to-time. We live in a harsh world, and we'll never be able to fully avoid pain and suffering. Regardless, I want you to always focus on the positive. When you do, you'll see a world of possibilities for your future, including your ability to move forward after your trauma.

Similarly, when you begin to focus on all the good things in your life, you'll see all that you have to be grateful for. Practicing gratitude daily has been a game changer for me. I spent many years in my teens and twenties wishing I were dead. Now that I'm on the other side of the devastation, I'm able to find joy all around me. I'm grateful for the littlest things because I'm still here to experience them. However, it took consistent practice on my part to train my brain to look for the beauty in every moment. I encourage you to also practice gratitude. Trust me, the rewards are most definitely worth it.

As the late pastor and motivational speaker, Dr. Myles Munroe said, "You cannot rise above the plane of your mental conditioning.

To change your life, you must change your mind."[13] The purpose of the next activity is to teach you to accumulate the resources that will help you change your mindset. When you're focused on the negatives about yourself, your life, and the world, it'll be difficult, if not impossible, to reach your goal. A negative mindset will always point out all the reasons you're going to fail, or why you're not deserving of the success. However, when you focus on the positives about yourself and the world, you'll be more open to new possibilities for yourself. You'll be more resourceful, and you'll see that you have options and the ability to achieve anything you set your mind to.

The next activity will teach you to use resources that are uplifting or cheerful to fight off negative energies. You could start or end your day with these resources, and you could use them throughout the day when you're feeling down. You could also use them whenever you have the desire to use a negative coping strategy you're trying to replace. You want to have the resources at the ready so whenever you need a shot of positivity, it's there. You want to develop an instinctual energy to fight off your inner critic as soon as it rears its ugly head. Like a fire extinguisher, you don't want to wait to get it until there's a fire blazing in your kitchen. You want to already have it and know how to use it before it's needed. I'm asking you to build your list of resources and practice using it before the fire (the overwhelm or sadness) consumes you. It's the only way your mind will default to use them when you're overwhelmed or feeling down.

Activity

By now, you should have already started collecting YouTube videos in different playlists. If you haven't created a playlist for motivation and inspiration, I encourage you to do that now. As a reminder from Chapter 2, you can sign up to receive my YouTube playlists as well as other recommended resources at serotinouslife.com/help. If you're not familiar with motivational and inspirational speakers, it'll give you a good place to start. You'll be able to see what messages resonate with you.

Next, I encourage you to create a YouTube playlist of videos that will make you laugh. I titled my own playlist "Laugh". You could search for "hilarious videos", or "funny clips", or "videos that will make me laugh". As you find videos you like, save them to your "Laugh" playlist. I also recommend you create a folder on your phone or computer with the title "Laugh" or "Smile" or both. I have one of each on my phone. I find that the images that make me smile elicit different feelings in me than the images that make me laugh. I don't always want to laugh before I go to bed because I feel more awake afterward, but I do like to smile before I go to bed. So, I'll often look at my folder of images that will make me smile while I'm lying in bed, right before I get ready to go to sleep.

As you come across quotes or images on social media you like, you can save them to your phone or computer. You can either save them directly to the folder you created, or move them to the appropriate folder right after you save them so you don't forget.

I'm confident that the more you fill your mind with positivity, and your time with smiles and laughter, the easier it'll be to tame your inner critic and replace your limiting beliefs with positive ones. You'll become more receptive to new ideas and ways of thinking, and your positive mindstate will increase your chances of reaching your goals and get you farther and farther away from the person you were and the life you had after experiencing your trauma.

Chapter 7
Ask for Help

I still struggle with depression from time to time. Whenever I tell my family and friends that I've had a few rough days, they always ask, "Why didn't you call me?" What they don't understand is that it's not instinctual for me to do that. Although I've gotten better at reaching out to my sister Nicole, or my mom, I still try to wait until I think it'll be a convenient time for them to talk. I'm so worried about inconveniencing them. This is definitely part of the overfunctioner in me, which I mentioned in Chapter 1. I try to so hard to be strong and independent so I don't burden anyone with my problems. However, it comes with a great cost. I still need other people. We all need other people.

As I've said before, humans are deeply social creatures. However, when we experience trauma, particularly at the hands of others, it makes us less likely to be vulnerable with others, in fear of being hurt again. This is why after Stan died, I got two cats, Sophie and Molly, which I still have today, 14 years later. I craved connection, but I was retreating away from humans. Not only was I continually hurt by the hands and words of humans, but I got hurt when they left me. I needed a break from the pain. Although my cats have become like my children and I'm immensely grateful for their companionship, I knew I needed more. Over the past few years, I've made a committed effort to improving the relationships in my life with the people who've proven to me time and again that they care about me.

It was difficult for me to emerge from my broken shell. Even though years had passed since my traumas, the memories are forever etched in my mind and I still carry the pain in my body. I had to admit that I was vulnerable and scared of getting hurt. I was very selective with who I shared this with. It was only with women who had stuck around for years, telling me time and again that they were there for me, even though I continually tried to push them away. The results have been nothing short of astonishing. The more vulnerable I became with them, the more vulnerable they were with me. I could see the beauty that could emerge when trusting another person. It made me want to keep going.

My friend, JoLynn is one of these women. I met her when I first started teaching in August 2009. We're both generally happy and bubbly, even though we've both experienced an immense amount of pain. She was always patient with me, and she could understand why I retreated at times because she herself had experienced pain. She was so understanding when I told her that I was working on improving my relationships, but I was scared. Over time I became more comfortable telling her when I was struggling instead of just retreating to my shell.

Soon after I published my first book in June 2021, I experienced a severe bout of depression, which was embarrassing because I just published a book about transforming after trauma. Luckily, I shared what I was going through with JoLynn, and she reminded me of the immense progress I've made in my journey. She told me that struggling with depression doesn't make me an imposter, and she reminded me that there will always be hard days even after experiencing great wins. She even gave me a Giving Key necklace that had the word "Faith" on it, which was given to her as a gift.

JoLynn wanted to provide me with a regular reminder to have faith that everything will be okay and I'll come out stronger on the other side. Of course, everything did turn out okay. It was just one of the many ways that life has tested me, like it does to all of us. Like all the passing storms in my life, I was shown once again that I could weather any storm and emerge with a little more strength and wisdom than I had before, in preparation for the next storm.

In his book, *Personality Isn't Permanent*, Dr. Benjamin Hardy discusses the importance of finding an empathetic witness that can help you process and think differently about your life experiences. He said, "You need people you can talk with openly about your struggles. You need people who can help you get to your own next level, otherwise you're going to get some emotional experiences, bottle them up, and plateau, or decline as a person."[4] JoLynn has become an important empathetic witness in my life. If you're guarded like I've been, I encourage you to seek out one empathetic witness to start. This person should be someone that can hold space for you, someone that will make time for you when you need them, someone that will be fully present with you when you're sharing your story, someone who won't judge you and won't try to change you.

My first empathetic witness was my therapist Patricia, whom I mentioned in the Introduction of this book. I never felt like she was trying to pull or push me farther along than I was ready to go. She walked alongside me, like a partner on my journey. It took a lot of trial and error to find her, but it was beautiful to find someone who could listen to my story and not try to push me through it quickly so they could avoid experiencing the discomfort of hearing my story.

Not everyone can be a good empathetic witness, even people who care about you. Think of how uncomfortable you've been during and after your trauma. When you're sharing your story, you transmit that discomfort to the listener, and not everyone can handle that. Most people's instinct is to push that discomfort away and resist more from coming, which is why many people will try to push you through your story and get you off topic so they can avoid feeling any further discomfort. The reason JoLynn is such a great empathetic witness is because, for years she's volunteered and worked with victims of sexual and domestic violence through various organizations. She's been trained how to listen to people's stories. It's also why my therapist, Patricia, is a great empathetic witness because she was trained to be so.

Unfortunately, not everyone who's been trained to be an empathetic witness is good at it, which is why I've had many undesirable experiences with other therapists. If you've had bad experiences with a therapist, family member, or friends, don't give up. It just means they're unable to sit with your discomfort. That's a reflection of them and not you. I want you to know that there are people out there that can listen to your story and not get scared away by it. Finding your own empathetic witness will take vulnerability on your part, and it may take feeling the sting of discovering people that can't be this for you, but the results will be powerful when you finally find a person that can be with you and your story.

Asking for help is a form of self-care. It's about listening to your body and mind and responding to its needs. This can be difficult after experiencing trauma, particularly if your trauma involved emotional, physical, or sexual abuse, or you continually question your role in the trauma and what you could have done differently. And since these experiences have taught you to not trust your instincts or caused you to doubt your instincts, it'll be difficult to learn to trust yourself again. But you'll get through it, and you'll learn to trust yourself again. Although it'll be difficult, it won't be impossible. I know from experience.

The next activity will help you take the first steps to asking for help. Once you begin to practice reaching out, it'll help bring down the guards you have against letting people in, and it'll be easier to listen to the internal wisdom your mind and body are trying to share. Over time, you'll begin to see that you're not floundering around the world on your own. By building a support network, you'll know that you have people to lean on and people that love you. Love is one of the best antidotes for emotional pain. You just have to be vulnerable enough to let people and their love in. It'll be hard, but you don't have to master it overnight. Just focus on continuously improving overtime. As one of my favorite mantras goes, "Bit by bit."

Activity

Get out our journal and write down the people that support you, love you unconditionally, and enrich your life. Also write down what their relationship means to you, and write at least one thing that they've done for you that meant a lot to you. Look at the list of people you wrote down and identify one or two people that you feel would be most supportive of your new goal and would most likely provide the support you'll need along the way. They'll become the foundation of your support system. These could be the same people you chose as part of your accountability team in Chapter 5.

The people I have as accountability partners aren't always the same people I have as my support system. They could be the same for you, but for me, they're usually different. There are friends and family I don't mind doing regular check-ins with, but they aren't always the same people I want to call when I'm having a hard day or I want to share exciting news with. Not every person in your life is going to be able to be everything for you. It's okay if some people are only there to share life with you on a superficial level, and others share your highest highs and lowest lows with you. They don't always have to be the same people.

Schedule a time to talk to or meet with the person or people you identified. When you talk with them, let them know how much you appreciate their love and support and how they enrich your life. I encourage you to remind them of the loving act they did for you that you wrote down in your journal. Even if you've previously told them how much you appreciate them, tell them again. Then tell them about the goal you're working on. Tell them why achieving this goal is important to you. Tell them that you know that achieving the goal won't be easy. Ask them if it would be okay to reach out to them from time to time to share your wins or struggles.

The next step is to actually reach out to them when you need it. I encourage you to practice in the beginning with reaching out to them with small wins, which includes just staying consistent with your progress. As you practice reaching out in the beginning, it'll become easier to reach out to them on your hard days. However, if you still find it difficult to reach out, ask members of your support system if they would be willing to check in on you from time to time if they haven't heard from you. Or you could ask them if you can provide them with updates on a regular basis, from once per day to once per week, depending on your goal. If it's a short-term goal or the goal is particularly challenging for you, you should check in more frequently. If it's a long-term goal or you feel like you don't need a lot of support, you could check in once per week. The check-ins will not only help you practice reaching out for support, but it'll also serve as an accountability system to keep you going.

If you feel like you don't have anyone to ask to support you, or you feel like you need additional support, I encourage you to consider finding a therapist or other trained professional. They'll not only support you but they'll also help you tackle the deep-seated wounds that are preventing you from getting close to other people and maintaining strong relationships. Although

I'm a strong advocate for us learning ways to cope with stress and pain on our own for the times when no one else is around, I also realize that we can't make it through life all on our own. If we try, it'll only lead to more suffering, even though suffering is exactly what we were trying to prevent by not getting close to people in the first place.

In addition to asking for help in the form of an emotional support system, you'll also need to practice asking for help in other aspects of your life. That's the purpose of the next activity.

Activity

Get out your journal and write down the areas of your life you could ask for help so you can dedicate more time and energy to reaching your goal. Do you live with other people whom you could ask to help with cooking, cleaning, and other household activities? Asking your family to start pitching in on household tasks may be difficult if they've always depended on you to do it. You'll need to have a conversation with them and explain why this is important to you. Write down who you'll need to talk to and prepare for the conversation. Think of objections they may have to your request and how you're going to handle those objections. Preparing ahead of time will prevent you from getting blind-sided by their objections. Don't take their objections as a reason for you to give up. Always remind yourself of why your goal is important to you so you can easily vocalize it to them.

Your loved ones deserve the right to voice their opinions. Show them that you value their feelings and what they have to say by listening without getting angry about them not supporting your goal. If you don't allow them this opportunity now, they'll likely try to sabotage your success consciously or subconsciously down the road because of unresolved resentments. Once they start helping you, it's important for you to find simple ways to show your appreciation, even if it's just saying, "Thank you."

Next, write down the tasks you could hire someone to do for you. Could you hire someone to mow your lawn, shovel the snow, watch your kids, clean your home, or do your grocery shopping? Also write down what you're going to do to make the money available to pay for this help. Although you can't foresee every roadblock on the path to achieving your goal, you want to anticipate as many as you can ahead of time. This way you can already have a plan in place to handle them. If you don't come up with a way to pay for this extra help ahead of time, the stress associated with finding a way to pay for it may cause you to want to give up or interpret it as a reason you won't succeed. You'll need to make sacrifices to reach your goal. This is where you'll need to remind yourself of what you said "Enough is enough" to in the Introduction of this book. You'll also need to remind yourself of your *why* that you discovered from the 5 *Whys* activity in Chapter 2.

Since I was a teenager, I've had the goal of hiring someone to clean my home for me. I've always disliked cleaning. I have family members and friends who find enjoyment in cleaning and see it as a way to relieve stress. I've tried to change the way I think about cleaning so I could view cleaning differently, but with each passing decade, my view on cleaning has stayed the same.

When I was getting ready to publish my first book and I saw all the energy I was going to need to put into marketing, podcast interviews, and social media posts, I knew something had to give. I work entirely from home, so it was distracting for me to look around and see everything that needed to be done. I just couldn't do it all. I couldn't clean, work a full-time job, run a business, exercise, maintain connections with my family and friends, and publish a book. I had also already started writing my second book (this book) while my first was being published. There just wasn't enough time in the day. I live alone, so I didn't have anyone else to ask to share the load with, so I had to pay to get tasks off my plate.

Although I had dreamed of hiring cleaners for years, when the moment came, I was scared to death. After experiencing numerous sexual violations, I became very protective of my space. My home became my sanctuary, my sacred space. I've always been careful of who I let into my home. I usually never let people in unless we have a close, loving relationship, and I trust them. Now I was looking at bringing complete strangers into my home once per week. Not only would they be coming into my home, but they would be touching my things and peering into all aspects of my private life. These thoughts terrified me.

As I got closer to the publication date of my book, and I could see the mounting obligations I had ahead of me, I began to feel overwhelmed. Everywhere I looked around my home, I saw tasks that needed to be done like vacuuming, dusting, and cleaning the bathroom and kitchen. Each time I looked around and saw all that needed to be done and knew that these activities would need to be repeated over and over, my heart sank further. I had to choose between moving through the discomfort of letting cleaners into my home and the discomfort of me doing the cleaning myself. Either way, I was going to be uncomfortable, so I had to choose which level of discomfort I was willing to handle.

Part of the work I've been doing with my trauma healing is to practice letting people into my life and space, particularly my home. During the few months leading up to hiring cleaners, I had started inviting friends into my home for the first time ever. Each time I asked a new friend to come over, I'd tell them that even though I care about them and I'm grateful for our friendship, letting people into my home is hard for me. Each friend was understanding and grateful that I was willing to share my sacred space with them. The practice of finally letting friends into my home, built up enough belief in me that I could also let strangers into my home and I would be okay.

Just like finding a good therapist took a lot of trial and error, finding a good, reliable cleaning service also took a lot of trial and error. Just like I wanted to give up on finding a good therapist, I wanted to give up on finding a good cleaning service because the process was so discouraging. But thankfully, I never gave up on either search. Not only did I find an amazing therapist but I eventually found an amazing cleaning service.

When I told my cleaners that letting people into my home was a big deal for me, they were very understanding. My cleaners have now become a cherished presence in my life. I not only trust them, but the work they take off my plate each week fills me with an immense sense of peace and relief. Instead of looking around my home stressing out over all that needs to be done, I look around and see a beautiful, clean home. I now smile when I look around my home instead of looking at it with a sense of dread over all that I need to do.

When I was deciding to hire cleaners, I knew I would need to make financial sacrifices. I had to remind myself that every time I say yes to one thing, I'm automatically saying no to another. This is the same for our time, energy, and money. In addition to not liking to clean, I don't like to cook either, so I used to eat out all the time. I would usually pick up at least one meal per day at a restaurant. When I thought about where the money to pay the cleaners would come from, I decided that I would stop ordering out and start making my own meals. Once I started doing that, I had all the money I needed to pay the cleaners. I also ended up with the delightful consequence of losing the extra weight caused by eating out. The sense of freedom I feel by taking the cleaning off my plate is worth every penny and every bit of inconvenience it's taken to make the money available to pay for it.

We all need help. None of us can do it all on our own. I know your traumatic experiences can make asking for help difficult and sometimes terrifying, but learning to ask for help and letting people in are part of the healing journey. The process will be bumpy and you'll get bruised at times, but keep going. The results will make every bump and bruise worth it.

Conclusion

Enjoy the Journey

It's so easy to focus on the final destination that you forget to enjoy the journey, but don't fail to enjoy the journey. Jim Rohn said that one of the great challenges of life is "being happy with what you have while in pursuit of what you want."[14] I found this to be true in my own life, especially when I first started climbing mountains. I climbed hundreds of mountains without ever taking a single picture. I rarely stopped to take in the surroundings. I just pushed to reach my goal (the top of the mountain) and tried not to focus too much on my physical pain on the way out. I did this until I began to hate hiking.

I started to dread going to the mountains because I wasn't focused on all the beauty along the way. I was so focused on my goals that I forgot why I fell in love with the mountains in the first place. I forgot that I got drawn into the mountains because they were where I first began to heal. They were where I first was able to see and embrace how strong I really was in both mind and body.

I began hiking when I was morbidly obese, so I was forced to regularly stop to catch my breath and take breaks. I was forced to take in my surroundings. I eventually lost weight and could go faster and farther without stopping. This excited me, so I wanted to keep going. However, I felt so strong that I started setting my sights on climbing some of the tallest mountains in the world. Eventually my hiking goals got so big that I couldn't stop. I had to keep going so I could challenge my body and mind for even bigger climbs in the future. Although I still love to push myself mentally and physically in the mountains, I'm much better at stopping and taking in my surrounding, taking pictures, and practicing gratitude for all that I have in my life.

Although I'm a huge proponent of reaching and striving for bigger goals, I also believe that you shouldn't treat goals as a way to escape from your current reality. If you do, you're bound to be disappointed. People always think their life will be different once they achieve a certain milestone, but once the dust settles and the excitement of the achievement clears, they're still left with the same person, doubts, frustrations and unhappiness they were filled with before. That's why it's important to find happiness where you are now, even if you're hoping for a different reality in the future.

I understand that some days are easier than others to make the choice to be happy in the face of anger, frustration, or sadness, but I find it troubling when I hear people say, "I'll be happy when I _____." The blank is usually filled in with so many different future circumstances such as, "I'll be happy when I get a new job," "I'll be happy when my kids get older and don't require as much of my time," "I'll be happy when I finish school," "I'll be happy when I get the big house, the big boat, the beautiful husband or wife," and so on. All I can think about when I hear people say these things is: "What happens if their goal takes 1, 2, 5, or 10 years to achieve?"

Does that mean they must wait that long to be happy? What happens if they never achieve the goal they were depending on for their happiness? Does that mean they'll be doomed to a life of misery? What if they get exactly what they desire and yet they still aren't happy? The truth is, if they can't be happy where they are now, it's unlikely they'll be happy when they finally get what they long for. Yes, they may experience happiness for a little while, but it'll fade away and they'll begin to feel miserable again, because they never changed how they were experiencing their present life. This is why I've been emphasizing changing your mindset throughout this book.

You must fill your mind with different inputs to prevent you from recycling old thoughts that are keeping you stuck in a place you no longer want to be. You need to change the way you're experiencing life right now, and the best way to do that is by changing your mindset and the way you think about your experiences. You must understand that reaching your goal is not most important, it's the person you become on the way to achieving your goal. By focusing intently on something that's important to you and removing the extra noise that will keep you trapped in old patterns, such as looking at people's lives on social media that make you feel worse about your own life, watching the news that fills you with fear, and engaging in idle chit-chat and gossip, you'll have more energy and desire to search for experiences in your life that reinforce that you're on the right path.

As you get rid of the things that take energy from you and replace them with motivational audio, personal development books, and searching for the beauty in every day, you'll have more energy and enthusiasm to pursue your chosen goal. And at the end of the day, it won't matter whether you achieve the goal or not, because as you're removing the toxic components of your life and instead focusing on giving your days meaning and purpose while simultaneously practicing gratitude for the simple blessings surrounding you in every moment, your life will be transformed. This will happen by taking the initial steps to change how you experience just one aspect of your life. The work you do to improve one aspect of your life will always trickle down and positively influence other aspects of your life. So embrace your small wins each day. Celebrate when you reach your goal, milestones along the way, or just the fact that you've avoided slipping back into old patterns.

I know all this probably sounds cliché, I know I'm ending on a flowery note, but I want you to know that you can achieve anything regardless of the immense suffering you've experienced in your life. You can choose at any moment to change the way you're currently experiencing life. That can begin my simply working to change one thing about your life. Not everything is going to change drastically overnight. Just like a huge ship can't turn on a dime, you're not going to be able to change every aspect of your life overnight. It'll take time, but all it takes is just deciding that you're sick and tired of experiencing life the way you currently are and deciding to make one change. As you do, you'll build momentum, you'll see how it's impacting your life, and you'll want to expand your reach into different aspects of your life. You'll begin to see that your trauma doesn't have to define how you'll experience the rest of your life.

I became empowered the moment I realized that I didn't have to keep cowering down in my life just because my victimizers tried to keep me small. They tried to steal my light but they didn't succeed. It took a while for me to unearth the little bit of light left inside of me after years of suffering. But the light has always been there. The more I focused on the beauty all around me, the brighter my internal light grew, and now I feel unstoppable. It took all that I had to endure and survive for me to realize that I can live life on my terms. I'm now living the life that my abusers never wanted me to have. I want you to also dig for that little light left inside of you. I want you to take a stand and say, "I want more from life, and I deserve to have it," because you do!

Acknowledgments

To my mom, Laura Lacey Curler, words can't begin to express how much I love and appreciate you. You've always encouraged the dreamer in me. You always made me feel that I could achieve anything I put my mind to, and you were always there cheering me on and ready to pick me up when I fell. Thank you for always loving me. That love has gotten me though my darkest days.

To my sister, Nicole, thank you for being there for me when I need to cry, complain, and celebrate. You have such a beautiful, loving soul, and I'm grateful for you every single day. I will forever cherish the special relationship we have.

Thank you to my editor, Emily Stark, for polishing my message and allowing my thoughts to flow better through the pages.

I want to say a big thank you to Jim Rohn and Les Brown, two of my most important mentors that I've never met. Jim Rohn's wisdom on business and living a great life are timeless. Les Brown's laughter always makes me laugh, and his words always move me to take action.

A big thank you goes to David Oliver, my business mentor and friend whom I met in the mountains. I find that very fitting, considering that I still go to the mountains to push myself and my beliefs about what's possible. David has pushed me to think differently about my business and helped me realize my vision of changing the lives of millions of people that are suffering in the aftermath of trauma. His willingness to tell me the truth even when he knew I wouldn't like it, has allowed my impact in the world to reach a whole other level. Thank you for believing in me and my mission.

I want to thank myself for not giving up. With every blow that life threw at me, I kept going. I'm proud of myself. It took me a long time to get to this point, where I want to shower myself with love and affection. So, I owe it to myself to put the words out to the world: I love me and everything I've done to survive.

To you who have been in that dark place where the suffering just seems like it'll never end, thank you for not giving up on yourself. Your commitment to stick with this book until the very end means that you still have that glimmer of hope inside of you. I promise you the darkness will end, but you must keep going. I'm very proud of you, and I believe in your ability to move forward. I wish you much success on your healing journey. You're worth every bit of it.

Lots of love,
Stephanie

End Notes

1. National Institute for the Clinical Application of Behavioral Medicine. (2021, October 4). *Successful ways to work with clients who struggle with deep feelings of shame.* [Online Course]. https://www.nicabm.com/program/shame/
2. Lechter, S. L., Reid, G., & Hill, N. (2019). *Success and something greater: Your magic key* [Audiobook]. Brilliance Audio. ASIN: B07W85XHQG.
3. Team Tony. (2021, October 19). *Discover the 6 human needs: These core needs drive every decision you make.* Tony Robbins. https://www.tonyrobbins.com/mind-meaning/do-you-need-to-feel-significant/
4. Hardy, B. (2020). *Personality isn't permanent: Break free from self-limiting beliefs and rewrite your story* [Audiobook]. Penguin Audio. ASIN: B08157LXPY.
5. Brown, L. (2020). *The ultimate Les Brown library: The Les Brown story* [Audiobook]. Nightingale-Conant. ASIN: B082Q68FD9.
6. Hopkins, T. (2018). *The official guide to success* [Audiobook]. Made for Success. ASIN: B07HHGBR9F.
7. Coelho, P. (2004). *The alchemist: A fable about following your dream* [Audiobook]. Harper Audio. ASIN: B000BO2D3C.
8. Esrick, M. (Director). (2019). *Cracked up: The Darrell Hammond story* [Film]. Healing from Trauma Film and Artemis Rising Foundation.

9. Morris, T. (2014). *The seven greatest success ideas: 'A-HAs' that are guaranteed to take your life to the next level* [Audiobook]. Nightingale Conant. ASIN: B00OH76WRW.
10. Chopra, D. (1999). *The seven spiritual laws of success: A practical guide to the fulfillment of your dreams* [Audiobook]. New World Library. ASIN: B0000548LZ.
11. Redfield, J. (2006). *The celestine prophecy: An adventure* [Audiobook]. Hachette Audio. ASIN: B000ENUXK0.
12. Maxwell, J. C. (2018). *Developing the leader within you 2.0* [Audiobook]. Harper Collins Leadership. ASIN: B0786ZNL3D.
13. Munroe, M. (2018). *The spirit of leadership: Cultivating the attributes that influence human action*. Whitaker House. ISBN: 978-1641230261.
14. Rohn, J. (2017). *The ultimate Jim Rohn library* [Audiobook]. Nightingale-Conant. ASIN: B076PQ4MTS.

Made in the USA
Middletown, DE
23 April 2022

64655518R00119